CURIOUS
POSES

For J and T, my microcosm

CURIOUS POSES

POSES

30 Yoga Postures and the Stories They Tell

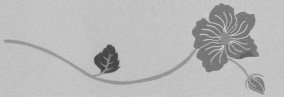

LUCY GREEVES

GREEN TREE

LONDON · OXFORD · NEW YORK · NEW DELHI · SYDNEY

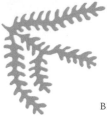

GREEN TREE
Bloomsbury Publishing Plc
50 Bedford Square, London, WC1B 3DP, UK
29 Earlsfort Terrace, Dublin 2, Ireland

BLOOMSBURY, GREEN TREE and the Green Tree logo
are trademarks of Bloomsbury Publishing Plc

First published in Great Britain 2022

Typeset in Spectral by Austin Taylor
Printed and bound in China by Toppan Leefung Printing

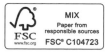

To find out more about our authors and books visit
www.bloomsbury.com and sign up for our newsletters

CONTENTS

INTRODUCTION

....

THIS IS A BOOK about 30 popular yoga postures, or *asana* – and what it might mean to strike these curious poses.

Did you ever catch yourself, halfway through a yoga session, thinking, 'Well, this is odd'? The first time it happened to me was during an outdoor yoga class about 15 years ago. A minute into a seated forward bend, I noticed that a tiny spider, the size of a pinhead, had started building a web between my calf muscle and my thigh. And in a moment of one-pointed concentration that ought to have been blissfully yogic, all I could think was what a very strange thing I was doing: sitting on a rectangle of rubber, with my body arranged in a specific and decidedly awkward set of angles, for a specific and seemingly interminable period of time, while a spider treated me like an interesting new tree stump.

It was like that feeling you get when you repeat a word so many times that it stops making sense: these shapes I had made with my body, probably hundreds of times over the course of each year, appeared suddenly in a new and baffling light. What was it really for, this arrangement of limbs? Why teach it like this, and not like that?

This curiosity fuelled me through three and a half intense years of teacher training, and 10 years of teaching yoga classes and retreats, and all the way out the other side to where I am today, investigating my questions in this book. Yoga is not the sort of terrain that offers a straight road from A to B; in fact, it's more like navigating a lush, overgrown jungle. But it is a fantastic generator of stories. Some of them are based on real events, and some are myths; some of them are metaphors, and still others are propaganda. The story of my own entry into yoga is a pedestrian one: I fell down the rabbit hole via an ashtanga yoga class (the fast, sweaty kind, with lots of jumping about) at a gym in East London, in 1999. My modest ambition, within these pages, is to map some of the meandering pathways that connect that moist, strip-lit room in a railway arch, full of Lycra-clad hipsters, all the way back to the court of the Maharaja of Mysore in the 1930s; the esoteric antics of New York high society in the Jazz Age; the blood-curdling feats of early modern Hindu ascetics; the mysteries of medieval tantric alchemy and the gnomic teachings of ancient Sanskrit literature.

As well as some of my favourite bits of yoga lore, both historical and mythological, I'll share observations and ideas for you to try in your own yoga practice. Yoga comes alive on the mat, when theory meets physical experience. However, this book is not an instruction manual: it doesn't lead you step by step into the poses, or list the risks and modifications that would allow you to practise safely in the absence of other guidance (which you should get ideally from a real live teacher). Think of it instead as a companion to your own explorations into the why, what and how of yoga *asana*.

Compared to the postures we assume in, say, a Pilates or HIIT class, the purpose of which we could describe as 'exercise' or 'body conditioning', the shapes of yoga *asana* feel loaded with symbolism. In many ways, the physical practice of yoga is more like a form of dance: a language of gestures that obliquely reveal their meanings. When we make these shapes with our bodies, we have the opportunity to do two things at once. The first is to absorb something meaningful from the experience, deepening our understanding of our own nature, and perhaps the nature of existence, too. The second is to communicate something meaningful – not necessarily to anyone in particular, but as an act of self-expression: a dance without an audience. The postures of yoga are multilayered metaphors that transfer meaning from the world outside to the world within us and back again.

The foundation level of that meaning is encoded in the postures themselves. Each of these special shapes is an exaggerated piece of body language. Reaching nobly towards the sky, balancing elegantly on one foot, folding deeply into a stylised bow: these are whole-body gestures that we instinctively understand to express a particular mood or emotion.

Next, the Sanskrit names of these postures point to a deep, rich layer of symbolic meaning. These names are sometimes drawn from Hindu scripture and mythology, sometimes inspired by animals, birds and plants, and sometimes by man-made objects like a gate or a bow. Over the course of centuries, the different branches and schools of yoga have woven in their own interpretations, until each *asana* is clothed in a delicately complex fabric of philosophy and symbolism.

For a long time now, yoga has also been an international affair. India has never been an isolated empire: long, long before the formation of the East India Company in 1600 (generally regarded as the first step towards British colonisation of India) its cities were busy hubs of multicultural exchange. As the writer and documentary filmmaker Gita Mehta puts it, 'At its best the culture of India is like a massive sponge, absorbing everything while purists shake their heads in despair.' During the first half of the twentieth century in particular, the physical practice of yoga underwent a period of rapid modernisation, as a result of which whole chunks of Indian classical dance, military fitness drills and Swedish gymnastics were folded into the postural canon. And as yoga has slowly grown to be one of India's most significant cultural exports, each new generation of international yoga devotees, tourists and confidence tricksters has added a patina of its own to the practices it either inherited, copied or stole (depending on who's telling the story). In recent years, the study of postural yoga has been enriched and complicated by insights from fields as diverse as neuroscience and psychology, anatomy and physiology, and even dance, anthropology and social justice.

And finally, there is you. Each time you move into your Crow, or your Lotus, you bring a new meaning to it. 'Deepening the pose' doesn't always mean tucking your foot behind your ear, or straightening your standing leg. Sometimes, it means unfolding a few layers of meaning, and allowing your own expression of the pose to blossom.

A note on Sanskrit transliteration

The Sanskrit alphabet has 46 letter sounds, which presents an English-language author with some challenges when trying to render it in our paltry 26 characters. With apologies to the purists, I have chosen to provide the closest available phonetic transliteration, without diacritical marks.

1
SITTING

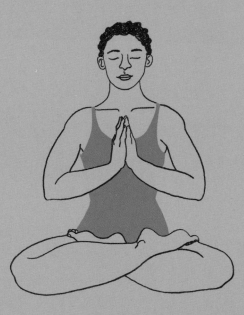

LOTUS POSE
Padmasana

....

AROUND 4,000 YEARS AGO, an unknown artist in the Indus Valley carved a stone seal that some people claim is the earliest surviving image of a yogin (student of yoga). It depicts a horned figure, seated on a small platform with his feet in front of him and knees out to the sides. Today, a similar cross-legged silhouette adorns herbal tea packaging and sports bottles around the world: Lotus pose has become the stock image for yoga.

IN CONTEXT

The lotus, *Nelumbo nucifera*, is the national flower of India. Its exquisite flowers, with their translucent white petals blushing to pink at the tips, can grow up to a foot wide. An aquatic plant that thrives in ponds and flooded fields, it is rooted in the soil but floating on the surface of the water and has been cultivated for its edible seeds for at least three millennia. It's said that an individual lotus plant can live for more than 1,000 years. But perhaps the most extraordinary thing about the lotus is its capacity for rebirth: in 1994, a group of scientists at UCLA successfully germinated a lotus seed from northern China dated at around 1,300 years old.

This beloved flower blooms abundantly in Hindu stories and scripture. The sacred text known as the *Shiva Purana* describes the time of the Great Dissolution, when all the objects of the world are dissolved into one undifferentiated ocean of potential. There is an intelligence here: Brahman, the eternal world-soul, pervades the void. It is immeasurable, incomprehensible, without form or name, but possessing the nature of pure knowledge, pure bliss. Despite its perfection, the being longs for another. Brahman wants to play. And so pure knowledge makes way for manifest beings. Shiva comes first, then Shakti, the male and female principal deities. Shiva decides it would be nice for someone else to get all the work done so that he and Shakti can concentrate on frolicking in the forests of bliss so he summons Vishnu into being, whose job is to make the world, protect it, and eventually dissolve it so that the whole divine game can begin again.

Vishnu lies down on the ocean of pure existence and falls asleep for a long time. As he sleeps, a huge and beautiful lotus flower grows out of his navel. From among its petals a new deity is born: Brahma, the four-headed god of creation. He is confused by his own sudden appearance: 'Who am I? Where did I come from? What is my duty? Whose son am I? Who created me?' Filled with existential questions, he begins to climb down the stalk of the lotus.

Brahma climbs for 100 years without reaching the base of the lotus stem. Then he begins to climb up again, 100 years without an answer. Eventually, after many more centuries of strife and suffering, he finally knows himself well enough to fulfil his destiny and create the world.

Whether or not the cross-legged figure on the Indus Valley seal is actually a yogin, *padmasana* is unquestionably one of the oldest yoga poses. The Sanskrit word *asana*, which came to be used to describe all the poses of hatha yoga, literally means 'seat'. And for the first 1,000 or so years of yoga practice for which we have textual evidence, it implied just that: a seated position for meditation. It's not until around the tenth century that complex balancing postures appear in the literature and standing poses come much later. From the beginning, stillness is a defining feature of yoga practice. Refraining from outward movement or action, and cultivating the cessation of mental chatter, is seen as profoundly purifying. Through these stilling practices, the yogin attempts to stop and even reverse the damaging accrual of *karma* – a richly complex concept, which in this case we can think of as a sort of existential

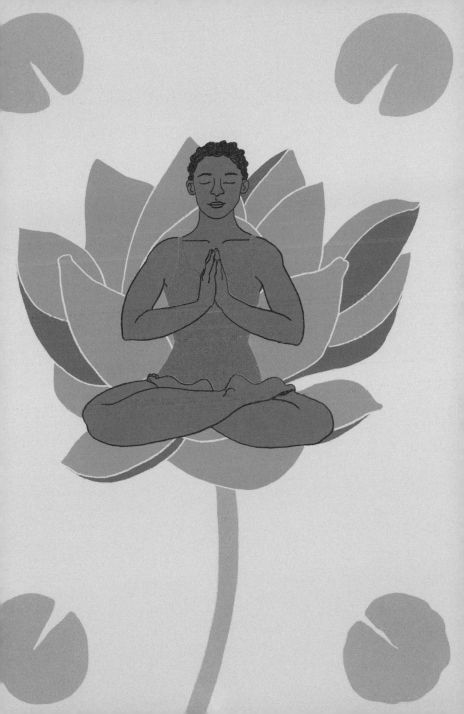

'rust' that builds up over our lifetimes, keeping us stuck in cycles of rebirth and suffering.

Because it has such a long association with the spiritual side of yoga, and because so many images use it as shorthand for blissful contemplation, and – to be honest – because it's difficult and therefore feels somewhat exclusive, *padmasana* is often spoken of as the pinnacle of physical yoga practice. But to see achieving 'full Lotus' as a goal, or the lotus as a symbol of enlightened perfection, is to miss the best part of the metaphor. Vishnu's lotus is a flower full of creative potential: the bud that unfolds its petals to reveal the very beginning of the world. But it's a world that is always in progress, never complete. Wander up and down the lotus stem for 200 years and you still won't reach enlightenment.

The lotus's ability to put forth pristine flowers while rooted in the mud of the riverbed is a lovely metaphor for our efforts to grow towards enlightenment out of the depths of our earthly attachments. So, approach the Lotus pose with an attitude of generous unfolding and be prepared to always be climbing towards a perfect flower that's just out of reach.

IN PRACTICE

'Place the right foot on the left thigh and the left foot on the right thigh.' The *Hathayogapradipika* (the foundational medieval yoga practice manual) makes *padmasana* sound simple. And if you're built like a fifteenth-century Indian ascetic, perhaps it is. Sitting cross-legged from childhood is a good start, but you also need slim legs and a high degree of flexibility in the hip joints. If you do happen to have that body type you might find *padmasana* an admirably steady, upright position that's ideal for meditation. But if, like me, you grew up in a world full of chairs and chocolate rather than crossed legs and lentils, even years of diligent practice may not be enough to attain this pose with any comfort.

To explore the lotus flower as a symbol of becoming, using

a *mudra* (hand gesture) can be a beautiful alternative to the full, pretzel-legged Lotus pose. It's worth noting that there's a text dating from around the eighth century that lists Lotus among a dozen different options for seated meditation. After that list, the author suggests a thirteenth option, a pose called *yathasukham* – which translates as 'whatever is comfortable'. As the Buddhist proverb has it, 'May you be like the lotus, at ease in muddy waters.' So, sit comfortably, with a straight back and legs relaxed, using whatever support you need to feel really stable. Bring your hands together in 'prayer position' in front of your heart, then relax the hands so that the palms separate but the heels of the hands and fingertips are still touching (this is your lotus bud). Soften your face and allow your eyes to close. Take a few deep sighing breaths to release any tension. As your breathing settles, begin to expand the lotus bud on each in-breath, keeping the heels of the hands touching but letting the petals of your fingers reach gently out and up towards the sun. On each out-breath, allow the flower to gently close and return to its resting bud.

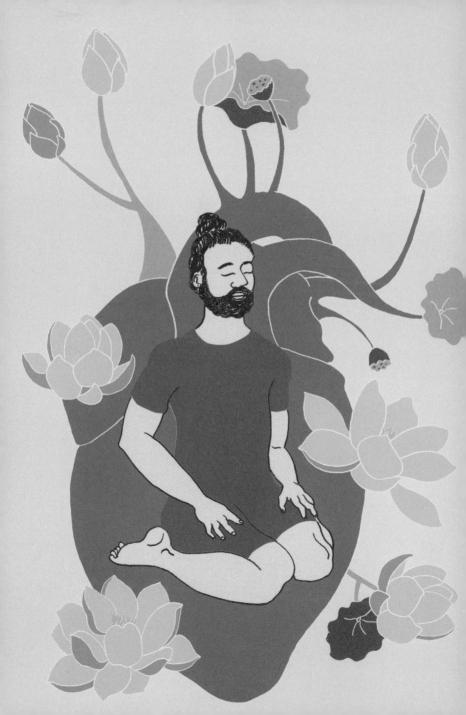

HERO POSE
Virasana

....

THE HERO POSE is a kneeling position. It's sometimes depicted with one foot folded underneath the hips and the other flat on the ground, so that one knee is up and one down, and sometimes with the sitting bones rooting down into the ground in between the folded legs. But it's always a quiet, contemplative attitude. In stark contrast to the powerful, expressive Warrior, the Hero is still and at ease.

IN CONTEXT

Virasana is one of the older yoga poses inasmuch as it's described in a number of the early hatha yoga texts. It's one of several postures associated with Hanuman, the monkey-faced *mahavir* or great hero of HIndu mythology. Hanuman's feats of strength and bravery at the head of his monkey army enliven the Hindu epics. He leaps across the bay of Lanka with a single stride, embarks on a perilous quest to bring back sacred herbs from the Himalayas, and slays a whole army of demons. All of this heroism is in service to his master, Lord Rama, at whose feet he is pleased to sit. And it's in this attitude of watchfulness and devotion that the Hero's pose finds him, folded on his knees.

What does it mean to be a hero at rest? Heroism is usually something you prove by deeds of courage and feats of strength, or perhaps an act of great sacrifice. With this pose, we are asked to take the heroism on trust. Great on the inside, ordinary on the outside. There's a beautiful passage in the *Chandogya Upanishad*, a dialogue between teacher and pupil, elegantly (if rather freely) rendered by Purohit Swami and W.B. Yeats like this:

> – In this body, in this town of Spirit, there is a little house
> shaped like a lotus, and in that house there is a little space.
> One should know what is there.
> – What is there? Why is it so important?
> – There is as much in that little space within the heart, as
> there is in the whole world outside. Heaven, earth, fire, wind,
> sun, moon, lightning, stars; whatever is and whatever is not,
> everything is there.

CHANDOGYA UPANISHAD 8.3.1–3

Ideas of macrocosm and microcosm – in this case, the big wide
world reflected in the smaller world of the body – are central to
both Vedic philosophy and tantric mysticism. And the notion of
a Tardis-like shrine inside the heart – a lotus room where you
can safely place the most precious object of contemplation, or
the whole chaos of the universe, or the unfathomable totality
of human consciousness – is a recurring theme in the esoteric
anatomy of yoga. Sometimes its dimensions and physical location
inside the body are described in precise detail, but it's also a
metaphysical place – call it a metaphor with coordinates. The
Chandogya Upanishad goes on to say that what is in that space
is eternal and does not decay or die with the body. That space
is the 'city of Brahman', the home of the essential self, free from
sin, old age, death, bereavement, hunger and thirst. In other
words, the central self of each individual shares in the nature
of the ultimate reality, Brahman: the universal consciousness
from which all the differentiated aspects of our material reality
emerge. And because its nature is one-ness and absolute truth,
this microcosmic self inside you is the source of both your
yearning for what is true and your dedication to learning it. Like
a homing beacon, it draws you back to yourself. Stop looking

elsewhere for the real thing, because it's all here. Infancy and old age, beauty and horror, emptiness and boundless bliss; the monkey and the hero.

Exploring yoga philosophy and symbolism can get a bit *Alice in Wonderland*: you're often asked to believe six impossible things before breakfast. I think it's crucial to bear in mind that these contradictions are a feature, not a bug. The puzzle presented by this *Upanishad*, the riddle of the universe inside your heart, works a bit like a Zen *koan*: it's a question without an answer, an invitation to practise with paradox. And it's designed to wake you up to something extremely disconcerting. Approaching the true nature of reality, according to yoga, is a bit like going to your front door and finding that it suddenly opens into outer space. I think the author(s) of the *Chandogya Upanishad* would have been pleased, but not surprised, to learn that astrophysicists now believe that our Milky Way galaxy is centred around a super-massive black hole and at its heart is a singularity: a one-dimensional point that is both infinitesimally small and four million times heavier than our sun.

IN PRACTICE

Hero pose can make a useful alternative to cross-legged seated positions. It's a resting posture for contemplation, so no outward heroics should be necessary. If your knees and hips protest loudly at the rotation necessary to sit the pelvis down between your ankles, keep the heels tucked underneath you in the closely related Diamond pose (*vajrasana*) or raise the hips with blocks or cushions to alleviate pressure on the joints. If it's uncomfortable to extend the front of your ankles flat along the ground, a rolled yoga mat or blanket underneath the ankles will help.

Hero pose is a moment to rest in your potential and come home to the mighty stillness at the centre of your gyroscopic being. It's a pose I like to put into a yoga session at least twice: once at the beginning, to notice what's going on and start to focus inwards, and then again towards the end, when the expansive effects of breathing and moving with attention may have changed my experience of being in my body.

Kneeling quietly, notice the space outlined by your ribcage and get curious about how it feels. Settle your attention towards the centre, where your heart is (you might even be able to sense or hear it beating). Allow your mind to go slightly out of focus and perhaps you'll notice that there's a place, there or thereabouts, where your attention can soften and rest. As your inner sense comes out to play, it might start riffing on sensations of bigness and smallness, finding all sorts of multi-dimensional space in between the delicate origami of your tissues. Did you know that the total surface area of your lungs – the epithelial layer through which respiratory gases are exchanged for air – is more than 50 square metres? Or that your body is home to over 60,000 miles of blood vessels – enough to circle the globe more than twice? Perhaps it's not surprising that we're sometimes inclined to feel bigger on the inside than on the outside.

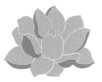

LION POSE
Simhasana

THIS POSTURE IS SOMETIMES called 'Lion's Breath' because there's a forceful exhalation that's integral to its execution. It is normally practised from kneeling, with the hands on the thighs or tucked beneath. Take a breath in to prepare, then move the chest and head forwards, sticking your tongue out forcefully and allowing your eyes to cross as you breathe out with a 'haaaaah!' sound.

Yes, from most objective standpoints, you do look ridiculous. Also, you are ferocity personified: pure wrath, unencumbered by notions of morality or decorum. This is the same expression found on the faces of Aztec jaguar masks, Chinese dancing lions and European cathedral gargoyles. It's an attitude that may well turn your enemies to stone.

IN CONTEXT

If asked to name an Indian big cat, most people would go for the tiger. But there was a time when the Asiatic lion was equally revered and considerably more widespread. By the late nineteenth century, it had been hunted almost to extinction – by both British 'sportsmen' and ruling-class Indians. Today, the entire wild population of Indian lions – fewer than 700 of them – can be found in northern India's Gir forest, where they have been protected by law since 1900.

The Asiatic lion is ferocious, wild, dangerous – in fact, anything but ridiculous. And as in real life, so in myth. Take the fearsome Narasimha, whose name literally means 'man-lion'. With a human body and a lion's great maned head and claws, he is an avatar created by Vishnu in order to defeat the evil demon Hiranyakashipu. This malevolent creature was persecuting Vishnu's followers and generally causing havoc – upsetting the course of *dharma*, the proper order of the universe. But his powers were so great that he could be defeated neither by night nor day, man, god or animal, inside or outside, on the ground or in the sky, and by no earthly or divine weapon. In order to solve the riddle of this demon's invincibility, Vishnu incarnated as the man-lion Narasimha – neither man, god or animal. Then he killed Hiranyakashipu at twilight (neither night nor day), on the threshold of a courtyard (neither inside nor outside), by putting him over his knee (neither on the ground nor in the sky) and disembowelling him with his lion claws (no earthly or divine weapon). *Dharma* was restored and the religious persecution of Vishnu's devotees ended.

Statues and paintings of Narasimha often depict the scene of Hiranyakashipu's death in grisly detail: the man-lion's jaws gaping in a ferocious roar, the surprised demon bent backwards over his lap, guts spooling out in a riot of scarlet. Sometimes, Narasimha is shown wearing the demon's intestines like a garland of flowers around his neck. Narasimha has at least nine other iconic guises, most of them equally terrifying. For example, there are sculptures of angry Narasimha, ferocious Narasimha, and Narasimha emitting the flames of wrath. But among all these fierce and forbidding personae, there's also yoga teacher Narasimha. Seated in meditation, his eyes are closed, his teeth hidden and his mighty talons folded into a *mudra* signifying peace.

Soon after I began my yoga teacher training course, I celebrated my 34th birthday. The same friends who, a year earlier, had given me, say, bottles of champagne or fun vintage earrings, turned up with herbal tea. And teapots, tea strainers, teacups: altogether, I counted eight separate tea-related gifts. It was as though everyone had got a memo that I definitely didn't send. I mean, I like herbal tea about as much as the next yoga teacher, but it's never been my 'thing' in the way someone might be into plane spotting, or

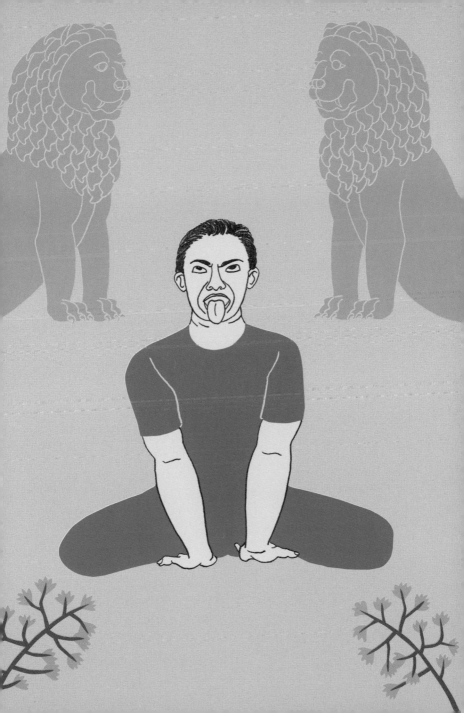

collecting china tortoises, or needle-felting portraits of Yorkshire terriers. It's just something I drink a few times a week. But in the minds of my friends, a sort of panicked gifting short circuit was occurring. Yoga teacher training = overnight interest in herbal tea. A yoga teacher, they were suggesting, is a person whose most intense celebratory pleasure is a nice cup of chamomile and spearmint, loose leaf, proper cup and saucer.

Me? I missed the champagne.

I fully understand the expectation that every yoga teacher should be a shining example of physical and moral fitness. I still feel a little shocked myself when I spot a yoga teacher sneaking a quick cigarette on the way to the studio. Yoga teachers feel compelled to hide their bad habits and even their injuries – especially those related to their yoga practice. We have to maintain the fiction that the teacher is winning on all fronts, that yoga does indeed confer a glowing superiority in mind and body – or risk undermining students' confidence in the thing we're selling.

Perhaps it's bad for business, but speaking as a student I'd prefer honesty over hypocrisy every time. I love the idea of lion-headed yoga teacher Narasimha, fierce and ridiculous and always straddling the edges of things, trying to keep one foot in each camp. Demon-slayer in the day job, pussycat in the yoga studio. I'm sure I'd learn something from studying under a living saint, but to date my most valuable teachers have been pragmatic and honest about the juggle of balancing the discipline of yoga with the demands of work and family life, and realistic about both the transformational powers of the practice – and its limitations. They've found humour and fellow feeling in the trying and the failing and the trying again. And they've shown me that getting past the performance and into the messy realness is the lion's share of the job.

IN PRACTICE

One of the nice things about doing yoga at home – whether self-directed or as part of an online class – is the feeling that nobody is watching. It's easier to make room for the ridiculous fierceness of this pose when nobody is looking at your lion face. But you know what? Nobody is looking at it during a studio class, either. In a world of face-tuned selfies and compulsive counting of 'likes', it can be salutary to remember that, most of the time, absolutely nobody is looking at you or thinking about you at all. Nobody. And yet – you still exist. You and your cross-eyed, fire-breathing, inner lion-person add up to a real entire thing, now and always, independent of the gaze of others.

So, wherever you are, take a few lion breaths and please feel free to really put some welly into it! Embrace the overlap between 'fierce' and 'ridiculous' and you might find the whole thing wildly cathartic.

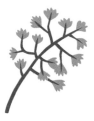

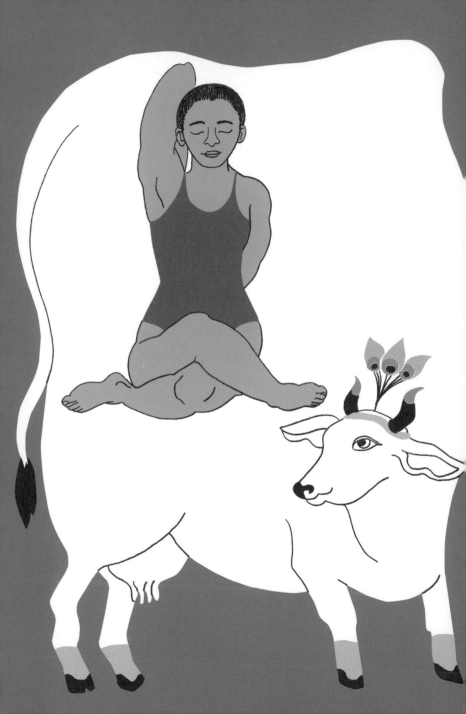

COW FACE POSE
Gomukhasana

....

FROM A SITTING POSITION, fold the left knee and bring the foot around to the outside of your right hip, allowing the bent knee to rest in front of you on the ground. Now fold the right knee and step over the bent left leg to bring your right foot alongside the opposite hip. Your knees will be stacked more or less on top of one another. Now lift your right arm up and, bending at the elbow, drop the right hand down between your shoulder blades. Reach the left arm behind your back to link hands in the region of your upper back. From above, your body's outline now mimics that of a cow's head. (Sort of.)

IN CONTEXT

It's time to take on the original sacred cow. She looms large in modern India, where to harm or kill a cow is taboo for most Hindus. This prohibition dates back a long way, to at least the first century CE; the milk-producing mama cow was already a special and sacred creature in ancient India and it's likely that the influence of vegetarian Buddhists and Jains was the final push that outlawed the consumption of beef.

Patient, devoted and above all generous, the cow appears in Indian scripture and epic as a sort of all-giving mother. In the ancient Sanskrit religious texts known as the Vedas (some of which date back as far as the second millennium BCE), the cow is associated with Aditi, the mother of all the gods. The fourth-century Hindu epic poem the *Mahabharata* contains an episode in which King Prithu threatens the Earth with his bow and arrow in order to force her to yield nourishment for his people. The Earth takes the form of a cow and begs him to spare her life, promising to provide enough milk and butter to feed everyone. It's a neat allegory for the transition from hunter-gatherer to pastoralist society and positions the cow as the sacred gift that keeps on giving – as long as she is treated peaceably.

The usual story is that Cow Face pose gets its name from its aerial silhouette – the stacked knees make the cow's nose, the feet its horns, while the looped arms create its flopping ears. But for me, the cow part is definitely reinforced by the low mooing sound that arises spontaneously every time I ease myself into the pose. Almost everyone who embarks on an exploration of hatha yoga eventually finds their nemesis pose, and *gomukhasana* is mine.

I don't hate it, exactly. It's just very far outside my comfort zone. For those of us who find it challenging, Cow Face pose can be exquisitely intense. A lot of this is to do with the construction of your hip joints: depending on the angle of the 'neck' of your thigh bone (femur), and the relative size of the ball and socket, you may find it easier to inwardly rotate your thighs (think knock-kneed) or externally rotate them (bow-legged). Cow Face pose is a particularly fiendish external rotator, because unlike the more natural seated external rotation in Cobbler's pose (with knees splayed out to the sides), it simultaneously asks that you adduct your thighs (cross them over each other). This adds a seriously spicy stretch across all your buttock muscles.

Love it or hate it, very few people are on the fence about *gomukhasana*. If it's not your nemesis then it's probably one of your favourites. During my teacher training, I used to watch open-mouthed as one of my peers casually folded herself into this pose for meditation sessions. It's hard to look at someone doing something that you can't do without mooing and believe that they are not just comfortable but downright relaxed – but there she was. I quickly realised that she and I simply had different bones. If I practised the pose a lot it might get a tiny bit more comfortable, but it was never going to be my jam.

IN PRACTICE

So, once you've identified your nemesis pose, is this something that you (as a diligent student of yoga) should avoid, or do more of?

These days, you'll often hear yoga types telling you to listen to your intuition. Sometimes it's characterised as heart wisdom, or the feminine principle: something body-centred, warm and emotional. I think the emphasis on intuition is in some ways a valuable corrective after decades of dominant guru-type yoga teachers, who encouraged their students to override their felt sensations in order to submit to the pose, or the practice. Many practitioners and teachers are making a conscious choice to centre bodily autonomy and end the long, harsh tradition of 'no pain, no gain' in yoga teaching. It feels liberating and necessary to celebrate the long-underestimated 'soft power' of gut feelings and trust your body to tell you what's safe and nourishing. But I find that when taken to extremes, the concept of yogic intuition can edge into something decidedly less healthy. The 'feminine principle' gets spiced up with exotic notes of Orientalism and set in binary opposition to the intellect, which is painted as masculine, Western, colonising, hard, arrogant, cold: in short, a real party pooper. By tuning into our inner wisdom, we're supposed to follow our bliss, towards love and away from judgement. Less head, more heart. Good vibes only.

But if I practise exclusively according to what feels intuitive and easy, I won't ever change much about the status quo. Just as when I try to avoid all the 'bad vibes', I end up staring at my own navel while blaming everyone else for the view. 'But wait,' I hear you say, '*my* intuition is different. My intuition also tells me to do hard things.' Well, that's lovely for you and I definitely believe you. Keep up the good work. For me, doing hard things requires something other than intuition to come into play. Call it willpower, call it discipline, it's a function of intellect and its job is to temper my intuitive tendency to take the safer and easier route. Intuition and intellect are not opposites, they're partners.

When I fold my body into the likeness of gentle, patient mother cow (oh, the irony!), my willpower has to negotiate an uneasy alliance with the sinews of my body, which are intuiting – hard – that a nice comfy Hero pose would be vastly preferable. It's a sticky, uncomfortable conversation with myself, and one that really wakes me up. I don't believe a body ever learns good things through pain and punishment, but nor does much growth occur without discomfort. So where is the point at which productive sensation tips over into pain? Where do I push, where do I hold back? This is yoga performing one of its most important functions: as a supercollider for false binaries, smashing my intellect against my intuition and humbling them both.

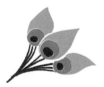

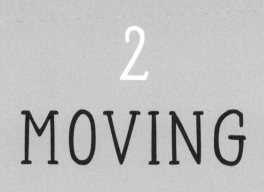

2

MOVING

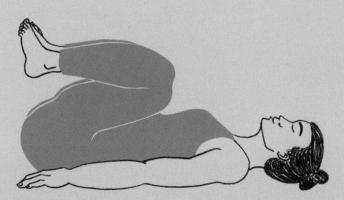

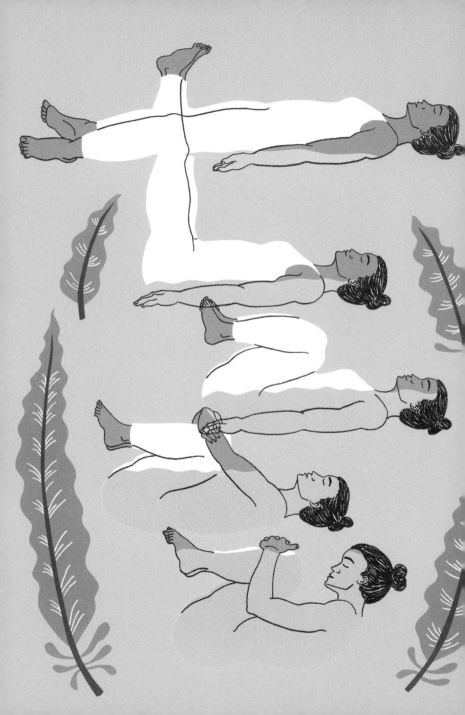

PRELIMINARIES
Pawanmuktasana

....

CALL ME CONTRARY, but my favourite part of a yoga practice isn't the flowing poetry of a Sun Salutation, or the exhilarating achievement of a headstand, or even the deep release of *savasana*: it's the warm-up. The bit that doesn't contain any recognisable poses. The bit that isn't really 'yoga' at all, except that it totally is: it's the necessary ritual that unlocks the gate to yoga.

The process of opening a gentle conversation with each part of my body and my nervous system becomes more precious to me as I grow older. I watch my mind starting to get quiet and my awareness sinking deeper down, as though I'm inching my way into a cool body of water. Everything else – to-do lists, nagging regrets, that increasingly familiar feeling that I've forgotten to put something on my to-do list, and that I'll regret it later – gets left on the mossy bank. Those things belong to a land-dwelling version of me and right now, I'm floating free of it all.

Achieving this state-shift, from mammal to amphibian, requires just the right level of preoccupation with the practice. Simple, repetitive movements that score low on technique and high on exploration work best for me. There should be a good number of them – enough to induce a state of reverie that's quite closely related to boredom. And they should follow in an intuitive sequence, ideally easing out each major joint in a row from head to toe, or vice versa.

IN CONTEXT

In traditional hatha yoga, this type of preparatory sequence is prescribed not just to free up the movement of the joints, but to release blockages in the body's subtle energies. According to the esoteric anatomy of yoga, our bodies are animated by a substance called *prana*, broadly comparable to the East Asian concept of *chi* or *qi*. *Prana* comes in different flavours, which move around the body as a series of *vayus* or 'winds'. These currents of energy closely interact with the physical breath, but are not the same thing. Maintaining an easy, balanced flow of *prana* is not just seen as good for your physical health; more importantly, it's essential to your spiritual progress. Most of the original hatha yoga techniques, and many that came later, are explicitly designed for pranic management.

The *pawanmuktasana* sequence (from *pawan*, a variation on *prana*, and *mukta*, to release), is a useful example. The first section begins with simple rotation of the ankles, then the knees and hips, then wrists, elbows, shoulders, neck – progressively limbering the joints and drawing you into that oh so soothing, almost-boredom state. The second section of the practice concentrates on the abdomen and digestion – lifting, lowering and tucking the legs, twisting through the belly. There's just enough concentration and effort required to call your mind back to the present moment without creating too much stress. The third and final section is a cathartic series of dynamic twisting, churning and chopping movements aimed at shifting energy blocks in the subtle body. On a good day, the whole set of movements leaves your nervous system humming like a finely tuned engine, your body engaged but free of tension.

Looking at the outward physical form of the poses, you can see how the whole sequence could be stripped of its esoteric elements and repackaged as a gym-friendly joint mobilisation, core strength and cardio class. Pop on a pumping playlist, get someone toned and upbeat to count out the movements like a pastel drill sergeant and put in about 10 minutes' work on branding – let's call it Praniacs™ – and we'd have an eminently franchisable wellness concept on our hands. But although I'd definitely still feel some benefits from the physical movements, I'm not sure it would have quite the same 'refreshing forest pool' effect on my nervous system.

When you're working at a psychosomatic level, intention matters. I'm not suggesting you have to buy wholesale into the notion of *prana* or energy knots to make this warm-up into a yoga practice (rather than a workout), but the intention to pay attention, to get quiet, turn inwards and be in conversation with yourself – that's non-negotiable.

IN PRACTICE

In the preliminary stages of a yoga session, you might think of yourself as a potter wedging clay or a baker kneading dough. The floor is your work surface and your body is the raw material you're working with. You need to compress and stretch it in skilful combinations to kick-start the internal processes that will result in a sound pot or a well-risen loaf. It helps if your movements are unhurried but rhythmic.

It's tempting to freestyle it completely – to 'listen to the clay' and let your body dictate what feels luscious for the muscles and freeing for the joints. However, I find that if I have no structure to follow at all, it's easy to zone out and just end up in a protracted warm-up (i.e. rolling around on the floor) for the whole of my practice time. There's nothing wrong with that experimental, stream-of-consciousness sort of vibe – it's a totally legitimate practice format. But for days when you want your yoga session to have some kind of narrative arc, a more structured warm-up sequence is more likely to set you up for success.

For me, counting repetitions is the key. Eight times on the right, eight on the left. Eight breaths clockwise, eight anticlockwise. Couple that with a simple, joint-by-joint sequence, working through the body from top to bottom or vice versa: you could learn the *pawanmuktasana* series, copy the opening 10 minutes of your favourite yoga class, or make up your own – it's not rocket science. That way you'll come to a definite point when you're done warming up and it's time to get down to some Proper Yoga.

SUN SALUTATION
Surya Namaskar

....

THE SUN SALUTATION that forms the basic scaffolding of the ashtanga vinyasa school of yoga is one of the most curious of poses. You may sometimes find yourself wondering, as I have done, whether you're in fact engaged in a very fancy sort of burpee: stretch up, hands to the ground, jump back, do a press-up, jump forwards, stretch up – but make it yoga. And if so, you might have hit upon an interesting knot in the tangled history of yoga and gymnastics.

IN CONTEXT

It's almost certain that the family resemblance between *surya namaskar* and a burpee is not just coincidence. The great hatha yoga modernisers of the first half of the twentieth century – Tirumalai Krishnamacharya and his star students, K. Pattabhi Jois and B.K.S. Iyengar – developed their practice with reference to a range of influences from both European and Indian physical culture. (This fertile period of cross-pollination has been well documented in recent years – if you're interested in digging deeper, key figures in contemporary English-language yoga scholarship for this period include Dr Elizabeth De Michelis and Dr Mark Singleton.) In later years, Krishnamacharya claimed that his method was derived from an ancient yoga text, which had conveniently been eaten by ants. But although sequences of yoga poses are present in the textual record from around 200 years earlier, the type of fast-moving sequences he pioneered at Mysore in the 1930s were clearly understood at the time as an innovation, and one that borrowed heavily from

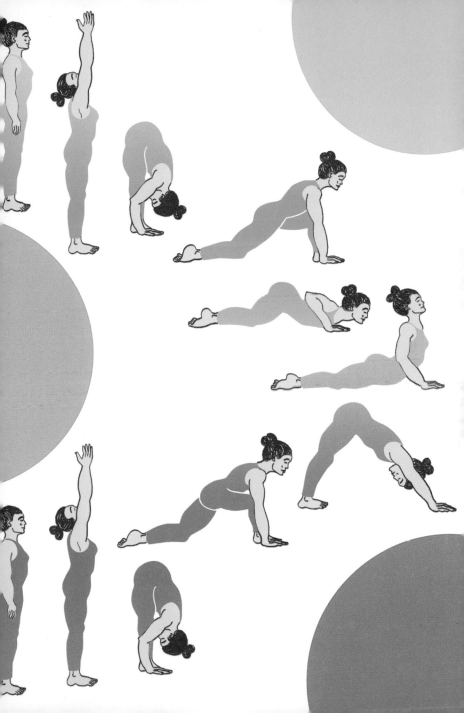

forms of gymnastics and body-building that were popular in India at that time; so much so that at least one of Krishnamacharya's contemporary critics accused him of promoting circus skills rather than yoga.

Anyone who has observed a taught ashtanga class in progress, in all its swooping, strenuous grace, knows that it's a beautiful spectacle. To the hypnotic soundtrack of synchronised *ujjayi* breathing (a technique to extend the length and refine the quality of the breath, which makes a characteristic 'Darth Vader' sound), the students stretch and fold and jump and float, in unison, through a precise series of poses and linking movements known as *vinyasa*. This perpetual motion yoga looks very different from the more traditional hatha yoga *asana* – long-held seated or balancing postures in which the primary discipline is endurance rather than agile movement. But they have something in common: both can be understood as a kind of performance – yoga as spectacle.

It's fashionable nowadays to talk of postural yoga as a type of inner work from which the outer appearance of the pose is an active distraction. The implication is that yoga-as-performance is not 'real' yoga. Whichever side of that particular argument you find yourself on, it's important to recognise that performance yoga is not a modern phenomenon. A very long time before Instagram, people liked to marvel at the strange things that yoga practitioners can do with their bodies. There's a centuries-long tradition in India of physical austerities as a devotional practice. Holy men became famous for feats like holding one arm up in the air, or standing up 24 hours a day, for months or even years. When pioneering spiritual tourist Theos Bernard travelled to India to learn hatha yoga in the 1930s, the main focus of his training was on posture duration: holding a headstand for a minute longer each day until he could stay in place for three hours at a stretch (*see also* p.91). Obviously, many if not most devotees practised their headstands in private – the fifteenth-century *Hathayogapradipika* specifies a secluded hut in the forest for the perfection of yoga *asana* – but having eschewed possessions and traditional forms of labour, the yogins still needed to eat. Displaying their skills in the public square in exchange for alms was extremely common.

The Sun Salutation – and by extension, the whole ashtanga vinyasa method – may also owe its format in part to the demands of public performance. In the 1930s, a young Pattabhi Jois was part of an elite troupe of young yogins trained by Krishnamacharya to demonstrate the more impressive aspects of hatha yoga to large audiences all over South India at the behest of the Maharaja of Mysore.

IN PRACTICE

To identify the rich stew of cultural influences that helped to shape *surya namaskar* is in no way to diminish its mysterious power and beauty. It wouldn't be the basic back-beat of (at a guess) half of all global yoga classes if it didn't move us deeply, scratch some kind of itch that our bodies have to stretch and move together. To flow through a dynamic yoga sequence as part of a group, with shared purpose, is an uncanny experience. Like a flock of starlings or a shoal of anchovies, each body is attuned to its neighbours. Moods and impulses can flit across the group without warning. Sometimes this group energy feels like solidarity, sometimes like competition. It can be expansive and exhilarating: can carry you through a tough practice that you would easily have given up if you were attempting it alone and take your practice to new levels. It can also drown out your interoceptive voice and take you beyond your safe physical limits. Likewise, compulsive repetition of Sun Salutations can be immensely soothing and can also open the door to repetitive strain injuries.

This group dynamic is a relatively recent innovation in yoga practice, which for the previous 1,500 years had always been a rather solitary pursuit, so I think it's interesting to compare how your Sun Salutations feel when you're alone in the room. It's a bit like exchanging the collective discipline of orchestral music for the looser explorations of jazz. Following that metaphor, you might like to experiment with tempo: how insanely sloooowly can you move through the sequence? Or go *andante*, each movement strolling smoothly into the next with no pauses. Or extemporise around the basic refrain; maybe even linger in one shape for the equivalent of a self-indulgent 10-minute drum solo.

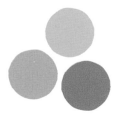

3
STANDING

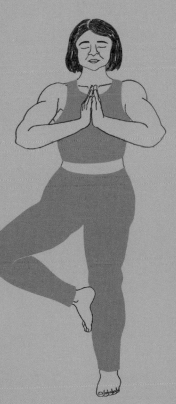

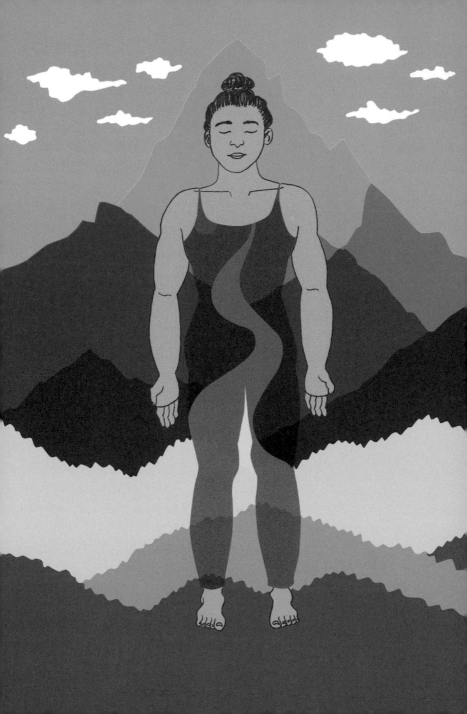

MOUNTAIN POSE
Tadasana

....

ALONG THE NORTHERNMOST border of present-day India, the great peaks of the Himalayas stand with their heads in the clouds, birthing sacred rivers. According to Hindu mythology, these peaks are mere foothills to a great golden mountain that forms the axis of the world. Mount Meru stretches down into the ground as far as it reaches up into the heavens.

Mountain pose, *tadasana*, evokes this mighty axis. Standing tall, balanced between grounding into the earth and reaching into the sky, the yogin in Mountain pose embodies *sthira* and *sukha*: the twin qualities of strength and softness that are at the heart of the practice.

IN CONTEXT

From Mount Meru to Mount Olympus, from the Hill of Tara in pagan Ireland to Mount Hikurangi in Maori New Zealand: since the earliest dawnings of religious thought, we have recognised mountains as sacred places. We populated them with gods because they were essentially unknowable, too cold or steep or oxygen-deficient to be explored. Now that high-tech climbing gear has put even the loftiest of them within reach, other measures are sometimes required. Mount Kailash is one of India's most sacred peaks and the traditional home of Shiva, one of the three central deities in the Hindu pantheon. Climbing it is strictly forbidden and (officially, at least) no mortal being has ever reached the summit.

In the ancient hymns of the Rig Veda, among the oldest-surviving religious texts anywhere in the world, the great mountains of India are personified as divine beings. Later, they were fabled as the homes of powerful demigods called *siddhas*, and so it followed that the mountains were the ideal place for serious yogins to perfect their practice. Krishnamacharya, who is often called the 'Father of Yoga' for his role in popularising the practice, is said to have spent a period of study with some mountain yogins in the Himalayas. It became a key part of his personal mythology that he had brought these secret and sacred teachings down from the mountains. Mountain teachings are extra special because they are hard to access, available only to the hardiest and most determined of initiates – or so the story goes.

The Mountain pose offers us a different way of knowing the mountains – one that requires a lot less personal risk and no altitude sickness. It invites us to speculate on how it might feel to *be* a mountain. Immense, patient, immovable; counting time in millennia. There is no dividing line where earth stops and mountain begins, just ground that gradually becomes uplands, that merge into foothills. To be a mountain is to be part of the physical fabric of the earth, yet intimately acquainted with the sky. Made of clay, but reaching for heaven.

The notion that yoga poses should be a balance between opposing forces finds its most succinct and poetic form in the text attributed to the sage Patanjali, which is usually referred to in English as the Yoga Sutras. Probably compiled some time around the second century CE, it consists of 196 gnomic aphorisms, a handful of which touch on the nature of yoga *asana*. For example, *sthira-sukham asanam* – that's the entirety of Sutra 2.46, and arguably the most influential three words in modern postural yoga – translates as 'The seat (*asana*) should be firm/strong/stable (*sthira*) and comfortable/sweet/easy (*sukha*)'. The influence of Buddhism on Patanjali's thinking was significant and I think it's fair to recognise in *sthira/sukha* echoes of the Middle Way: neither punishingly ascetic nor prone to sensual indulgence.

Although Patanjali was talking about *asana* in the ancient

sense, as a seat for meditation, his advice holds good for the modern sense of *asana* too. The Mountain pose is about seeking that perfect equilibrium between reaching up and grounding down, where both forms of striving dissolve into simply standing, simply being. The point where effort and surrender, *sthira* and *sukha*, become a third thing: not what you're doing, but what is. The middle way is where you can gain clarity about your nature. It's not about 'me as mountain' or 'what mountain means to me', but rather about reaching far enough down into the dirt and up into the ether that in the end, the gods dissolve too and the fact of the mountain is enough. In the words of poet David Ignatow, 'I should be content/ to look at a mountain/ for what it is/ and not as a comment on my life.'

IN PRACTICE

Inasmuch as it's a close cousin to simply standing up straight, *tadasana* is more about a quality of attention than any special physical technique or effort. Stand with the feet roughly hip-distance apart, so that your pelvis is stacked squarely on your two thigh bones and your weight transfers evenly down through the knees, ankles and feet. Both footprints should feel steady and even, with the weight releasing equally down through left and right sides, heels and balls of feet. From the bowl of the pelvis, the axis of the spine can extend its long, springy natural curves upwards. The shoulder girdle rests easily on the cushion of the lungs and the head finds an alignment with the spine that feels almost weightless. All this is held up by the deep muscular structures of legs and torso, hugging the skeleton gently but firmly. You're looking for a steady, alert sensation of standing that is neither parade ground stiff nor bus stop casual.

Mountain pose offers the perfect opportunity for you to observe the interplay between strength (*sthira*) and softness (*sukha*). Watch out for unnecessary holding in the face: it's common for a certain amount of unconscious effort to happen in the jaw, tongue and eyes when you're concentrating hard. Is the belly soft enough for the breath to flow easily, or is the pelvic floor held and the ribcage braced? Is your gaze soft or staring? What's the least effort you can make to hold the shape and what's the most? Make a scale in your head, from least effort to most. Try dialling up and down until you feel you can identify a point of perfect equilibrium: that Goldilocks zone that's neither too soft, nor too strong, but just right.

TREE POSE
Vrikshasana

....

ON A MASSIVE GRANITE boulder at the UNESCO World Heritage Site near Mahabalipuram – a city on India's south-east coast, not far from modern-day Chennai – a man has been standing on one leg, with his arms stretched skywards, for almost 1,400 years.

He is the still centre of a stunning bas relief, over 25 metres long and 12 metres high, which depicts almost 150 near-life-size humans, gods, mythical creatures and animals. It's a masterpiece of rock carving, dating back to the mid-seventh century. Baby elephants, mocking monkeys and a sarcastic cat are among the more delightful details. The identity of the central figure, standing in what we now recognise as Tree pose, is disputed: is he the semi-divine warrior hero Arjuna, performing austerities in order to win the magical spear Pasupata from Lord Shiva? Or is he the sage Bharigatha, doing penance in order to call the mighty River Ganges down from the heavens?

IN CONTEXT

An earlier name for the balancing posture commonly known as Tree pose was *eka pada pranamasana*, which literally translates as 'one-legged prayer pose'. Like an entry in the ancient *Guinness World Records*, its mythos is built on feats of endurance: various adepts were said to have held the pose for 100 days, 12 years and – in the case of the Bharigatha legend – 1,000 years. Such austerities were the primary means by which to acquire *tapas*, a Sanskrit term that can be translated variously as austerity, ascetic power, discipline or heat. The theory was that physical penances were the best way to accumulate *tapas* and thereby burn away *karma* (the effects of your actions on Earth), thus allowing you to step off the wheel of rebirth and attain liberation. Among the 18 traditional penances described by eighteenth-century ascetic Puran Puri are a lifelong vow of silence, standing on your head on top of a betel nut, and the method he chose for himself: living for the rest of your days – morning, noon and night – with your arms held up above your head (he assured his biographer that the pain diminishes after the third year).

But for those of us not so religiously invested in burning up *karma*, where does discipline end and punishment begin? I know that at some point fairly early into the first hour of standing on one leg with my arms held up above my head, it would occur to me that I was harming my body and I would stop it. Take away the incentive of saving my soul from thousands of lifetimes of suffering and there's just pain without meaning. So I particularly welcome this pose's other name, *vrikshasana* or Tree pose, which seems to invite us to engage with a gentler form of asceticism. Trees don't punish themselves for 1,000 years, they just get on with being part of the forest.

Forests are special places for yogins, right from the start. Gurus sit under benevolent shade trees to give their teachings. Renunciates retreat to the peace of the forest to build their simple huts and practise yoga without disrupting the complex web of plants and creatures that coexist there. Because a tree is not just a solitary wooden thing sticking out of the ground: it's an organism completely in tune with the ecosystem above, around and underneath it. Leaves capture sunlight and turn it into sugar (I know, it's basically magic!). Branches and trunks give safe harbour to birds, insects and smaller life forms. Roots extend down into the earth, making space for moles and rabbits, then further through the ghostly web of fungi through which the whole forest stays in touch. These mycorrhizal networks allow trees to support their offspring, cooperate with allies and sabotage their rivals in a sophisticated community.

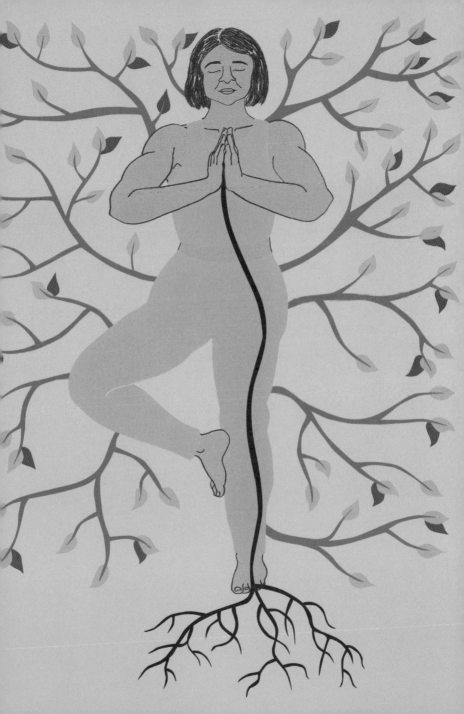

Maybe spending 100 days in one-legged prayer pose is one route to enlightenment. Perhaps it's even a route into the tree-ness of Tree pose: maybe, out on the other side of agony, there's a moment of knowing what it would feel like to be a different arrangement of carbon and stardust, one that we call wood instead of flesh. I'll never know. I'm putting my money on the possibility that the effort of empathy with a tree can come more softly, without requiring me to disown my own embodiment.

IN PRACTICE

Like so many aspects of yoga, Tree pose is an exercise in reconciling paradox. The student must become still enough to meditate, while also maintaining a precarious standing position that involves 50 per cent fewer legs than usual. For me, visualisation helps a whole lot: I imagine roots growing down through the floor from my standing foot and the organising logic of concentric rings of wood around a central core. I've got another secret, though: an accident of proportion means that my thighs and shins are exactly the right relative length to prop my bent leg comfortably against the standing thigh. It feels completely secure – a bit like clicking the leg of a folding table into place. There's no skill involved because it felt that way the very first time I tried it – it's just how I'm built.

We all have poses that 'make sense' for our bodies and others that really don't. If you weren't born with 'folding table' legs, maybe Tree pose will always be a conundrum for you, or maybe modifying it with some props (a block between foot and thigh, a wall behind you) will make more sense of it. Either way, don't worry about it – just be more tree. You are doing *vrikshasana* any time you are intentionally rooting downwards through your legs and growing upwards through your arms and torso, feeling the slow pulse of the forest.

MIGHTY POSE
Utkatasana

························

EVERY STUDENT OF YOGA sooner or later finds a pose that forcefully recalls its roots in the endurance feats of devout ascetics. If Tree pose doesn't do it for you, try a long hold in Mighty pose, *utkatasana*. It's a zigzag-shaped standing pose: flexing the ankles, bending the knees, hinging forwards at the hips as if frozen in the act of sitting down, with arms raised alongside the ears. Although often called 'Chair pose', it lacks cushions. It is rigorous, demanding, without frills – a hard wooden bench of a posture.

IN CONTEXT

As well as 'mighty', the Sanskrit word *utkata* can be translated as fierce, proud, superior, intense, awkward, difficult, out of the ordinary, or even frightening. To understand the distinctive flavour of this pose, it's worth diving a little deeper into the concept of *tapas*, which I touched on in the previous section (*see also* p. 47). *Tapas* is often translated as 'austerity', and it's a concept with a similarly chequered reputation.

If we go back to the beginning – or as far as textual sources will take us – we find *tapas* depicted as a powerful energy source: in the Vedas, the sun's *tapas* creates all life on Earth and the process by which men are transformed into sages is also described as *tapas*. The etymological root of the word is in *tap*, meaning to heat or burn. And like fire, *tapas* can be both friend and foe. Historically, ascetics known as *tapasvin* used extreme physical self-discipline as a route to enlightenment but there's also evidence (from the nineteenth century) that Indian schoolteachers used postures

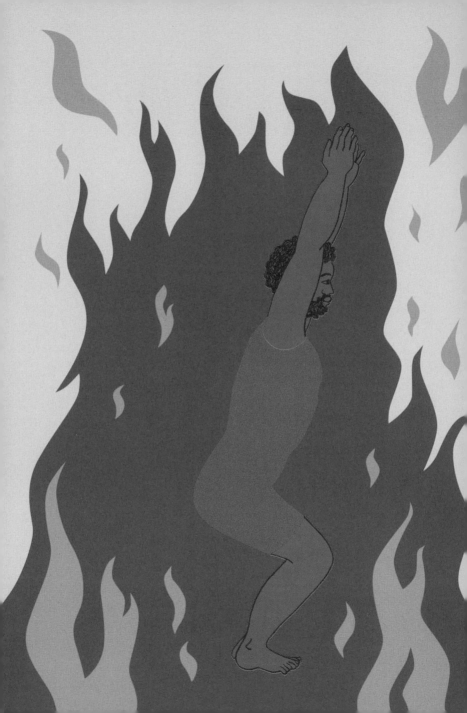

indistinguishable from yoga *asana* to punish naughty boys – I'm sure half an hour in Mighty pose would have left them feeling very sorry indeed.

Tough physical discipline was a feature of twentieth-century yoga schools, too. The 'Father of Modern Yoga', T.V. Krishnamacharya, was photographed literally standing on his young students during his public lectures, while the boys held exacting yoga postures. Both of his most famous students, Jois and Iyengar, told of beatings at Krishnamacharya's hands, which they seem to have largely accepted as a normal part of their training – the guru's prerogative. When B.K.S. Iyengar died in 2014, among the hagiographic tributes were some more qualified accounts of the great man. According to Malini Nair, an Indian reporter who attended one of Iyengar's workshops, 'Slouched spines get a shove, and lazy knees a sharp slap as the taskmaster is merciless in his quest for the perfect pose. I escape with a light but well-aimed kick to my recalcitrant left heel.' Iyengar's US students apparently used to joke that B.K.S. stood for 'beat, kick, slap'.

The yoga world has faced a series of reckonings in recent years. A long history of abuse has come to light, both physical and sexual, perpetrated by a depressing number of high-profile 'gurus' upon their students and staff. It's important for everyone who cares about yoga to hear and acknowledge the stories of these victims. It's also clear that detailing the many and various shames of twentieth-century yoga is beyond the scope of this book: writers far more qualified than me are doing this hard and necessary work elsewhere, applying some purifying *tapas* of their own to the task. But here and now, the sticky question remains: is corporal punishment simply baked into the hatha yoga tradition, or can these poses be mighty without being all-the-way frightening?

Through a modern lens, the concept of austerity still contains the dual nature of fire: it can be a terrible destructive force and a source of energy. On the one hand, we have austerity as government policy, intended to have a bracing effect on the poor by stripping them of frivolous 'luxuries' like heating, healthy food and a social safety net – all very energising if you're among the ruling classes, but devastating if you're at the bottom of the ladder. And on the other hand, we have 'austere' as an aesthetic choice that inspires calm and mental clarity – think minimalist interiors and stark architecture. Or austerity as a personal badge of honour, where intermittent fasting and cold-water swimming offer ways to wake up from the stultifying material comforts of late capitalism. Unadorned, stripped of pretension, radically plain and clear: something that's austere can also be exhilarating and deeply satisfying.

IN PRACTICE

As every hero knows, physical trials must be faced and overcome on the way to longed-for new states. Those of us who have given birth are intimately familiar with this idea, and I imagine the same is true for people who train for marathons or climb mountains. So let's hold in mind that the intensity of *tapas* is built into the yoga journey, and that its purpose is transformation. In hatha yoga, the term *tapas* is sometimes used to mean 'inner heat' – a metaphorical fire that has a tempering effect on the physical body, toughening and purifying. Many of the techniques and poses of hatha yoga are specifically aimed at increasing this heat: for example, the slow but fierce *ujjayi* breath (*see also* p.38), the abdominal contraction known as *uddiyana bandha*, and strong standing poses like this one. A minute or so in Mighty pose really does raise your body temperature – and sets your thighs on fire (a useful thing to know if you're starting your yoga practice in a cold room and need to warm up quickly!).

Although yoga is intimately concerned with stillness and balance, that state of equilibrium isn't achieved through simply stopping moving. We have to apply some forceful action first in order to get unstuck from our habitual patterns. In the *Bhagavad*

Gita, yoga is famously defined as 'skill in action': to be alive is to act upon the world, and the challenge is to harness that action skilfully enough that it becomes a route to greater self-knowledge and spiritual understanding, rather than a destructive dead end. When working with any poses that feel mighty or frightening, it's critical to develop an ability to tell the difference between forceful action in pursuit of greater clarity and forceful action whose end result is numbing, distraction or punishment.

Yes, Mighty pose can feel somewhat punishing. It can also feel exhilarating, empowering, and strangely comforting in its intensity. The difference is in your intention and the quality of your observation. Try getting really quiet in Mighty pose and notice everything that comes up. Here, my body feels stuck, but over here I feel strong. Round about now, I want to run away but I won't. Now it's time to go deeper – and now it's time to stop.

DOWNWARD-FACING DOG POSE
Adho Mukha Svanasana

....

THE CLASSIC Downward-facing Dog pose describes a right angle at the hips, supported by strong, straight arms and legs. Tail high, muzzle low: the canine inspiration for this four-legged pose is instantly recognisable. The proper name for this kind of natural doggy gesture is pandiculation, an involuntary stretch that's a bit like a whole-body yawn. For a bipedal human body, it's quite effortful to bear our body weight on our arms, so although we may mimic the shape of a dog's expansive morning stretch, we tend to experience it more as a pose of strength.

IN CONTEXT

The status of the dog in Indian society and culture is conflicted. The subcontinent is home to around 35 million stray dogs, living in close proximity to humans but not welcome in their homes. Since these strays spread diseases (including around 20,000 cases of rabies each year) and survive mainly on scraps scavenged from rubbish, it's not a stretch to understand why many Indians regard dogs as unclean and teach their children to fear them.

The most widespread semi-feral dog breed in India was commonly known as the pariah dog (following a recent rebrand, it's more sensitively called a Desi dog or INDog today). The word *pariah*, which we use in English to refer to a social outcast, carries a similar meaning in India; it comes from a Tamil word used to

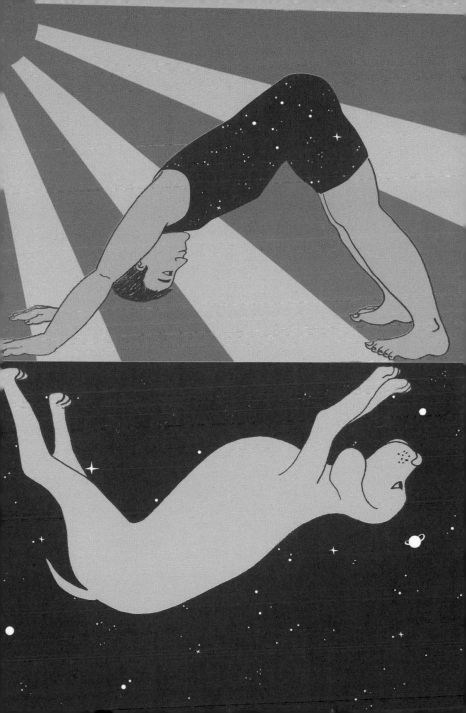

describe the lowest-ranking individuals in the Indian caste system. Likely a close match for some of the earliest-ever domesticated dogs, pariah dogs are smart, loyal and tough. They don't shed or drool very much and they're not as disease-prone as many pedigree dogs: in short, they make excellent pets. In recent years there's been a boom in street-dog adoptions in India, which has gone some way to improving the breed's outcast status.

Dogs in Indian mythology walk a similar tightrope between acceptance and rejection. In the penultimate book of the *Mahabharata*, the five semi-divine sons of King Pandu decide to renounce their earthly possessions and spend the rest of their lives practising Yoga in its fullest sense. The inevitable end of this spiritual quest will be death, welcomed as a release from the sufferings and illusions of this world. Accompanied by their collective wife Draupadi, and a nameless dog that decides to tag along, the five brothers set out to roam the world as wandering yogins. One by one, their vices become their downfall: pride, vanity, self-regard and boastfulness bring about the deaths of everyone except the eldest brother, Yudhishthira – and the dog.

At last, the thousand-eyed god Indra comes down in a celestial car and offers to transport him to heaven. But Yudhishthira refuses to go on without the dog, which by now has advanced several levels from opportunistic hanger-on to faithful companion. As the one surviving brother tells the god, 'This is my vow: I will never give up a person who is terrified, nor one who is devoted to me, nor one who seeks my protection because he is destitute, nor one that is too weak to protect himself.' Despite the god's remonstrations that dog owners don't get into heaven, and his escalating descriptions of the rewards the hero will get in exchange for going on without the dog, Yudhishthira stands firm. Suddenly, the dog is revealed as Dharma, the god of righteousness, in disguise. He congratulates Yudhishthira for having passed the final test and welcomes him into heaven.

The moral of this story – apart from 'be nice to dogs' – is that the practice of capital-Y Yoga requires you to reject easy rewards and pursue your moral convictions, sometimes to the point of contrarianism. Or, perhaps, that it pays to be empathetic and protect the vulnerable, even when that flies in the face of convention. From its origins among ash-smeared forest-dwelling renunciates to its hippie resurgence, to its current awkward straddle of New Age spirituality and exercise medicine, hatha yoga has always been a practice that hovers around the edges of the mainstream. At some points in time it has seemed to be approaching cultural and social respectability, at others very much not. In the Downward-facing Dog – part shanty-town stray, part Dharma in disguise – it has found a fitting mascot.

IN PRACTICE

In modern postural yoga classes, Downward-facing Dog is often used as a 'reset' in between flowing posture sequences or asymmetrical poses. Some irritating teachers will tell you it's supposed to be a 'resting pose', but that's just a power play. Some active muscular effort through the legs, arms and shoulders is important here, to manage the amount of stress on the joints in this deeply unnatural position, so don't worry if it feels like work.

You also need a lot of length in your hamstrings, openness in the shoulder joints and deep flexion at the ankles – none of them particularly natural to the average adult human. I think yoga teachers, most of whom have made this shape with their bodies literally thousands, maybe tens of thousands of times, tend to forget how weird it is. There is absolutely no reason why this pose should be easy – or even accessible – the first few hundred times around.

The key to Downward-facing Dog is getting your spine into what's called axial extension: in other words, a slightly extended and lengthened version of its natural, neutral curves. Your limbs are secondary, which means you can make whatever compromises are necessary, today, in your arms and legs so that your spine can express this extension properly. Start on all fours, making good contact with the mat through your hands and lower legs, and tune in to the whole length of the spine. Feel how it curves up into the upper back and down into the back of the waist like an elongated letter 'S'. Now tuck your toes under and imagine a gentle tug through the tail end of the 'S', straightening it out as your hips rise up and back. The weight of your head at the other end of the 'S' will help lengthen it downwards at the same time. Feel your legs begin to straighten and as soon as your tailbone starts to tuck under and lose the length in your spine, stop. Over time, you'll be able to work into straighter legs without losing the long, straight spine.

WARRIOR POSE
Virabhadrasana

....

THE WARRIOR SEQUENCE brings a flavour of martial arts on to the yoga mat. These are big, confident standing poses that can make you feel proud and uncompromising. They speak of decisive action: arms outstretched, making your presence felt in the world. In the first three versions of the pose, the feet are placed wide, with legs in a strong lunge. Warrior 1 stretches both arms to the sky, with hips and trunk facing forwards; Warrior 2 turns the hips and trunk to the side with arms outspread to front and rear, at shoulder height; the third variation, Reverse Warrior, lifts the leading arm aloft and sinks the trailing arm to add a backbend. In the final variation, Flying Warrior, the yogin moves into a one-legged balance, stretching both arms forwards and the lifted leg backwards.

IN CONTEXT

Virabhadrasana takes its name from a mythical warrior who personified the wrath of Shiva. Shiva is all about wrath: in his guise as the Destroyer he strikes down ignorance and wrongdoing, and is ultimately responsible for calling time on the universe itself. Despite his fearsome temper, his forbidding aspect – ash-smeared, dreadlocked, clad in an ascetic's loincloth – and his habit of retreating to the mountain tops to meditate for 1,000 years, he maintains a passionate partnership with Shakti, his feminine 'other half'. Their love is so strong, it persists through multiple incarnations. In one of these, Shakti is reborn as Sati, the daughter of a mortal nobleman named Daksha.

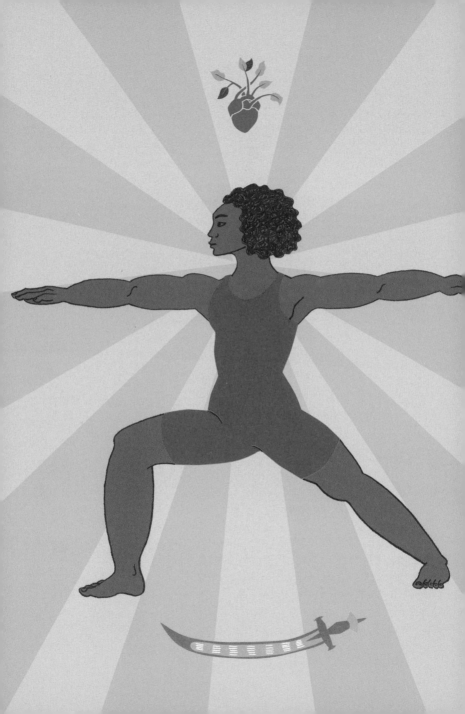

Perhaps unsurprisingly, Daksha disapproves of young Sati's relationship with the god Shiva. He tries everything he can to keep them apart and find a more manageable match for her but Sati won't be fobbed off with a dull human suitor. In despair at Daksha's attempts to control her, she sets herself on fire in the middle of a big festival and dies in flames. When word reaches Shiva, his anger overcomes him; he rips out one of his own dreadlocks and throws it down from Mount Kailash to land in Sati's ashes. At the very moment his matted hair meets her charred bones, the warrior Virabhadra springs from the ground, sword raised (Warrior 1). With a single sweep of his sword, he slices Daksha's head off (Warrior 2), holds it aloft to his master (Reverse Warrior), then brandishes the grinning trophy at the watching crowds (Flying Warrior).

Shiva is far from the only militant yogin. In the *Bhagavad Gita*, the famously conflicted warrior Arjuna takes a time out on the battlefield to debate the right course of action with the god Krishna. He's reluctant to fight against his many kinsmen and friends who have chosen to position themselves on the opposing side of the battle but Krishna urges him to 'kill with the sword of knowledge this doubt, born of ignorance, that has arisen in your heart. Take refuge in yoga and arise, great warrior.' The whole text is a meditation on spiritual struggle and the war on ignorance, but it's also a story that ends with Arjuna taking up his bow and going to fight with real weapons against his former allies.

We can trace the legacy of Arjuna's yogin/warrior nature on into early modern times. From around the fifteenth to the early nineteenth centuries, bands of ascetic yogins in India often worked as mercenaries: warriors for hire. They were seen as guerrilla fighters, countercultural figures who disrupted trade routes and organised effective military resistance to established rulers. Their activities were criminalised under British colonial rule and eventually suppressed by increased policing.

Despite this long history of martial yogins, the Warrior poses didn't form part of the hatha yoga repertoire until the twentieth century. Certainly, similar poses are found throughout Indian art as far back as 100 BCE, but they only became yoga staples during the 1920s and 30s. During this period, which coincided with India's struggle for independence from British rule, the development of hatha yoga in India was intimately concerned with questions of machismo and strength, and nationalist identity. Once again, yoga and militancy went hand in hand.

IN PRACTICE

The power of the Warrior poses comes from the way they fire up the muscles of the legs and hips, forcing a marriage of effort and stability. There's a sense of barely suppressed movement in the shapes, as though frozen in mid-stride. From the strong base created by the feet and legs, the torso can rise straight and graceful, with a lightness in the shoulders and arms. When all these elements work together in a yoga class, you can see people's faces become very still and serene. It's all a little unsettling when you think of Virabhadra coolly slicing off Daksha's head.

Decapitation or no decapitation, I absolutely love these poses and I love to teach them. The notion of yoga as warlike, let alone as an expression of militant Hindu nationalism, doesn't sit comfortably with modern, Western perceptions of the practice as a route to inner peace. It's a common workaround to reframe the bloody violence of the Warrior sequence's origin myths as a metaphor for spiritual warfare: like Arjuna, we wield a sword of knowledge and slay our enemy, ignorance. But in practice, these bold, provocative stances tap into something aggressive inside me that is hard to entirely sanitise as metaphor. It feels *so good* to stand proud and implacable, to inhabit a body that's fired up and weaponised.

'Do I really want to kill somebody?' I find myself thinking, as I shoot invisible yoga laser beams out of my fingertips. Probably not – or not right now, at least. But I do very much want to challenge those who overstep the mark and threaten my integrity. I do want to 'fight the good fight' and stand up for what I believe is right. And I want to get in touch with that masculine warrior energy: not to fear it, but to harness it and own it, so that it doesn't own me. It's not all love and light in yogaland, or indeed in the real world.

With the exception of the one-legged Flying Warrior variation, the Warrior poses are not normally classified as balancing poses. Nevertheless, they demand a strong sense of balanced effort. It's really common for people to 'front load' the poses, because our effort tends to follow where the gaze goes: when facing, and lunging, forwards, the back half of the body can trail off a little. See what happens when you deliberately transfer your attention (but not your gaze) over your shoulder to the back half of the pose and try to send equal effort and equal weight through the soles of both feet. Often, this brings a lovely feeling of centring, which transforms the energy of the pose from belligerent to coolly assertive.

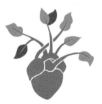

TRIANGLE POSE
Trikonasana

....

THERE'S SOMETHING of the Egyptian frieze about Triangle pose: the body turned to fit within a flat plane, describing sharp angles with its straight-line straddled legs, side-tipped torso and outstretched arms. Unlike Indian wall carvings, where figures crouch, kneel, sway hips and bend knees, seeming always about to burst out of their stone frames, *trikonasana* attempts to pin you to the papyrus in two dimensions.

IN CONTEXT

Although Triangle pose has become part of the modern postural yoga canon, there's no trace of it before the twentieth century. No ancient roots or mythological backstory – just an exacting but elegant shape to put your body in. It's also the gateway to a central debate in modern yoga: to align, or not to align? Try to shape yourself into a triangle and you're immediately confronted with the inconvenient truth that human bodies are not made up of flat planes or straight lines. Even the straightest bits – the shin bone, for example – turn out on closer examination to be full of tension and hidden spirals. Inasmuch as *trikonasana* is an attempt to mould our curvaceous organic matter into the clean lines of geometry, it is doomed to failure.

    Much modern-day difference of opinion among yoga teachers centres around the principles of alignment. Put simply, how much does the geometry of the pose matter? Trainee teachers learn (to a greater or lesser extent, depending on which school they follow) cues to instruct the students into 'proper alignment' in each

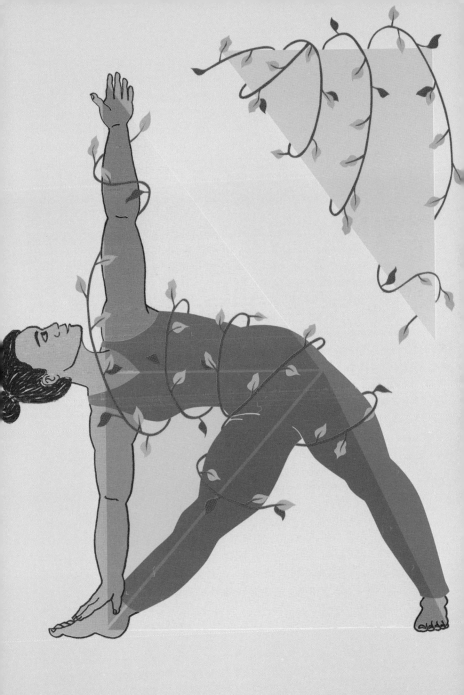

pose. These are often presented as safety requirements, to stop the injurious loading of a particular joint, or excessive strain on a ligament. But as anyone who has graduated to the point of teaching real bodies will know, observing and preventing such events is more complicated than simply telling students to keep the knee above the ankle, or place the heels in line. It takes some time of working with a particular student to really understand their angles, movement patterns, comfort zones. What feels unsafe in one body is an easy option for others. I'm not sure why this needs to be said, but I'll say it anyway: each body is different.

The spectrum of views on alignment runs from, at one end, the hyper-formalists as exemplified by B.K.S. Iyengar to the functional movement gang at the other. Iyengar was one of the great twentieth-century popularisers of yoga outside India. His book *Light on Yoga* has sold over three million copies in 23 languages. At the heart of the book is an extraordinary series of 600-odd photographs of Iyengar demonstrating yoga poses. It's a visual hymn to *tapas*, to the terrible beauty of physical discipline. Although his facial expression is serene, his presence hums with intensity: you can see just how hard he is working to make it look easy. As he himself put it, 'I have sweated and toiled in my gruelling practice, unmindful of the pain and suffering.'

A closer look at the pictures reveals an idiosyncratic body: Iyengar had a relatively short, barrel-shaped torso, slim legs with long shins, and strikingly long arms (standing in Mountain pose, his fingertips reach almost to his knees). Even setting aside years of rigorous training beginning in childhood, there are things this particular body can do by virtue of its conformation that will never be accessible to humans of a different build – and yet, thanks to this iconic set of images, Iyengar has become the Vitruvian Man of modern postural yoga: the template for all our Triangles, Mountains and Warriors. When we follow the precise alignment cues of his disciples, we are de facto trying to be shaped more like Mr Iyengar. Is this intrinsically helpful or necessary? Probably not.

Although if we are determined to strive towards an external model of postural perfection, perhaps one body makes about as much sense as any other.

Functional movement advocates, on the other hand, argue that if we discard notions of 'perfect' form or alignment and instead try to use and adapt the poses to reveal the intrinsic soundness of each individual body, then yoga can be reinterpreted as a therapeutic modality in the here and now (rather than a vehicle for salvation). Instead of moulding ourselves into 'ideal' shapes, we can work with the functional properties of our own joints and tissues to learn to live more comfortably in our bodies.

To a devotee of medieval hatha yoga – rooted in a tradition of motionless austerities and the belief that extreme physical discipline provides the energy necessary to escape the earthly cycle of suffering – I suspect this approach would seem too far from his understanding of the purpose of yoga *asana* to be accommodated under the same name. But as he mellowed into old age, even Krishnamacharya himself – the same man who stood on his students' spines and put them through punishing *vinyasa* drills (*see also* p. 53) – developed a far more adaptive, therapeutic style of yoga that aimed to adapt the pose to the individual, not vice versa. It's an important strand of teaching, harking back to the edict in Patanjali's Yoga Sutras (*c.* second century CE) that the yogin's pose should be both *sthira* and *sukha*: firm but gentle. And it informs a more compassionate approach to postural practice today. The latest alignment-sceptic yoga methods continue this tradition, seeking to integrate new insights about how our bodies move and thrive to make yoga more accessible and therapeutic for a wider range of bodies.

IN PRACTICE

To see how the alignment question plays out in Triangle pose, you can try it two ways. From B.K.S. Iyengar's *Light on Yoga*, observe the following blueprint: place your feet 3–3.5 feet (about a metre) apart, right foot turned out 90 degrees, left foot turned slightly to the right, legs stretched and knees engaged. Now bend your trunk sideways to the right, bringing the right palm towards the floor (stop with the hand on your shin if you can't reach the floor with straight legs). Stretch the left arm up in line with the right shoulder. Keep the backs of the legs, back of the chest and the hips in line. Come back out of the pose slowly and carefully.

Now try again, with the instructions proposed by Peter Blackaby (in his book *Intelligent Yoga*). An osteopath and functional movement expert who initially trained as an Iyengar yoga teacher before breaking away from the tradition, Blackaby recommends removing the side-bending aspect of the pose, which he says can create a damaging 'shearing' force across the sacroiliac joint at the base of the spine. In his hands, the posture is a forward bend with a spinal twist. Step the right foot forwards, then hinge forwards at the hips to bring the fingertips to the floor (or a block), just ahead of your right foot. Keeping the hips and legs steady and the spine long, rotate through the spine to turn the chest towards the left and stretch the left fingertips up towards the ceiling.

However you choose to practise it, perhaps the real point of Triangle pose is not to succeed in transcending three-dimensional reality and achieving trianglehood, but to learn something about the gap between the blueprint and the reality.

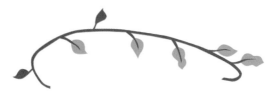

GATE POSE
Parighasana

....

GATE POSE IS NAMED for the Sanskrit *parigha*, a crossbar or beam used to shut a gate. From a high kneeling position, extend one leg out to the side with the foot firmly planted on the floor in line with the opposite knee. Press down through the 'standing' knee and stretch up the arm on the same side; come into a sideways bend by reaching the outstretched arm over towards the outstretched leg.

In this pose, your body becomes both the gate and the latch or bar that locks it. It's an invitation to reflect on what you allow in and what you exclude: to consider the body as a keeper of boundaries.

IN CONTEXT

The techniques of traditional hatha yoga are deeply concerned with boundaries. There's a whole set of practices involving *mudras* or seals, and *bandhas* or locks: gestures and contractions designed to help the practitioner to capture and contain energy inside the body. This underlines the fact that early hatha yogins are preoccupied with the body's role as a container for the breath and the vital energies – and good containers don't leak. In general, modern yoga teaching tends to downplay the containment side of things, instead leaning into an obsession with stretching: making the body more and more malleable and 'open'. Which begs the question, is there such a thing as *too* flexible? What would that look like, physically and psychologically, and what might we learn from it?

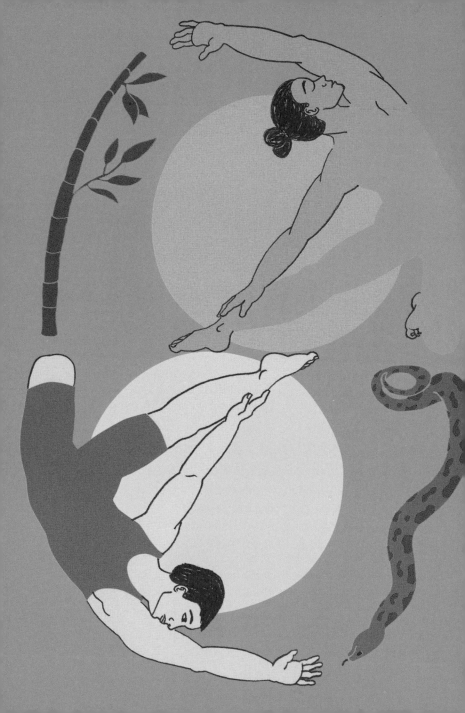

From a physical point of view, excessive flexibility shows up in unstable joints. When a joint is regularly pushed outside its healthy range of motion, the supporting ligaments can become lax and no longer support the action of the joint in the way they are designed to. We can look to individuals with Ehlers-Danlos syndromes – a set of conditions that affect the body's connective tissues, often resulting in hypermobile joints – to see the sort of challenges that come with excessive flexibility: joint pain, frequent dislocations, early onset osteoarthritis. These are extremes, of course. A far more common presentation in lifelong hatha yoga practitioners like me is a general, low-grade pelvic instability – which I suspect is caused or at least aggravated by years of studious devotion to lengthening the hamstrings.

So, one important boundary for yoga students to bear in mind is around how far you need or want to go into a pose: whether you're better served by lengthening and opening, or by strengthening and shoring up a particular joint. I once tangled with a teacher who was urging me further and further into a deep forward bend: 'What if my hamstrings are already long enough?' I asked. They didn't have an answer for me. I think the concept was so foreign to their training that they couldn't parse out the question, let alone come up with a response. In circumstances like this, you have to be ready to set your own boundaries.

The physical consequences of excessive flexibility are relatively obvious. I think the unseen psychological implications might ultimately be more pernicious. As an embodied philosophy, yoga has the trick of turning the body into a working metaphor for the mind. The goal is strong and flexible bodies, with strong and flexible minds. But when we emphasise yielding and extending and melting at the expense of grounding and resisting and consolidating, we risk becoming too flexible at the emotional/psychological level. We become liable to bend over backwards, to surrender too soon, to bow down when we should rise up.

I've touched already on some of the yoga abuse scandals

that have come to light in recent years. For me, the gathering momentum of yoga's own #MeToo movement has delivered some striking lessons about how the fetish for flexibility can obscure and enable the harms enacted by teachers in positions of power. The elements of the story may vary, but with depressing regularity, a powerful male teacher persuades thousands of devoted students that submission to the guru and the practice are prerequisites for spiritual advancement, that pain is a sign of progress – and that unsolicited hands-on adjustments from the teacher are to be welcomed without question. The emphasis on allowing the guru to *literally* bend the student into whatever shape he chooses seems designed to compound the imbalance of power and completely erase the victim's sense of agency.

But I also see the pitfalls of excessive flexibility play out in subtler, more everyday ways. I see friends of mine using mindfulness or yoga to develop that paralysing combination of resilience and compliance required to stay on indefinitely in a crappy job or a spent relationship – just as I have done at different times in my life. Perhaps you've heard yourself say something like 'This is a great exercise in sublimating my ego' or 'I just have to open my heart more'. Well, maybe. These are valid concerns. But sometimes we also need to stand our ground and bar the gate. Sometimes we need to take up the space we were born to occupy, instead of always trying to bend ourselves, soften ourselves, flex ourselves around other people's priorities.

IN PRACTICE

Gate pose is a great place to hang out and play with strength and flexibility. The lower body needs to be strong and steady while the upper body flexes, with a long stretch along almost the whole lateral line. You can feel the complementary impulses of strength (*sthira*) and softness (*sukha*).

If you're a flexible sort, you probably enjoy the feeling of reaching far into a stretch. It might be worth spending some time contemplating what you get from that. Is there balance in your practice, and in your life? If you were less flexible, what would you lose? What might you gain?

If you've always felt you are not flexible enough, or worried about the fact that you can't get into 'advanced' poses, contemplate those fears. What would it prove for you if you could do those things with your body? Are there good reasons for your resistance? Chances are you'll get a little clearer about where you draw the line.

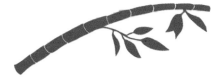

4
BALANCING

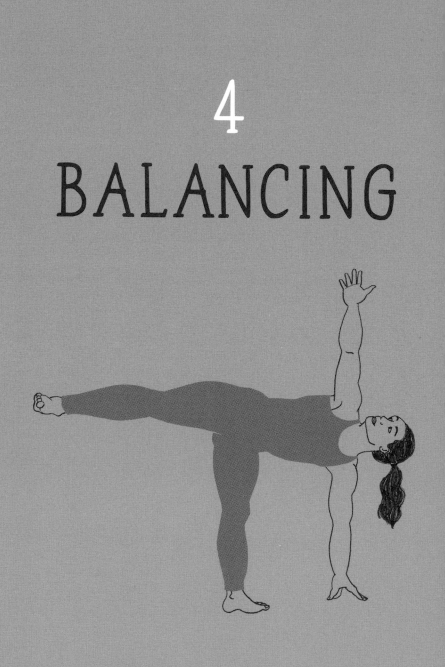

CROW POSE
Kakasana

....

AS BALANCING POSES GO, this one is straight in at the deep end; it's a fine test of overall strength and coordination, too. From a deep squat, place your hands on the mat in front of you, a little narrower than shoulder-width apart. Turn out the toes and nestle your knees tightly into the outside edge of the upper arms (triceps). Lifting up and forwards (look for a sensation of your heart rising into the space between your shoulder blades), allow your hands to slightly claw at the mat as you tip your weight gradually forwards on to the arms. Continue lifting up and forwards so that you can come on to tiptoes and finally to balance with the feet completely off the floor. Your arms become the legs of the crow, your legs its folded wings; your gaze follows your beaky nose down towards the ground in front of you – perhaps somewhat alert to the danger of toppling face-first on to your yoga mat.

IN CONTEXT

The *asana* most often referred to as Crow pose (*kakasana*) in the West is known more commonly in India as Crane pose (*bakasana*). Some say it's a Crane when you practise with the arms straight, a Crow with the elbows bent – but that's a hard one to adjudicate. So, are we Team Crow or Team Crane? I'm afraid I find the Crow altogether a more interesting bird, so with apologies to brother *baka*, that's where I'm going with this.

So, what is it like to be a crow?

Corvids are some of the most intelligent non-human creatures on Earth. They mate for life, live in complex social groups, make and use simple tools, and plan ahead to solve problems. Among the other cool things that crows can do: recognise faces, play in the snow, and drop hard nuts on to pedestrian crossings in order to use cars as giant nutcrackers.

Some biologists argue that crows aren't necessarily cleverer than other creatures, it's just that their mental abilities are more familiar to us than, say, echolocation in bats or the 'hive mind' of bees. Corvids are clever in a human way, and we flatter ourselves that represents the high-water mark for intelligence. But despite the similarities we intuit when we watch a crow figuring things out, we can never really know what it's like to *be* one.

At least, that's the proposition at the heart of Thomas Nagel's famous 1974 essay, 'What is it like to be a bat?' Nagel argues that the limitations imposed by the shape and scope of our own minds prevent us from ever truly entering into the consciousness, the point of view, of another intelligence. We can know every single fact about another creature – or even another person – and still not come close to apprehending what the world looks and feels like to them. Nagel says that 'such an understanding may be permanently denied to us by the limits of our nature... there are facts that do not consist in the truth of propositions expressible in a human language.' The closest we can come to the experience of bat-ness or crow-ness is through our imagination.

Through this lens, the Crow pose becomes a meditation on the nature and limitations of mind and body: how can I transcend the boundaries of my singular experience in order to enter into the experience of another, let alone dissolve into the ocean of pure existence? Perhaps the greatest balancing act in yoga is not perching the whole of your folded bodyweight on your hands, but holding in your mind the contradictions of being at once a bounded body and an intrinsic part of a single, unbounded consciousness. Reaching for crow-mind, and beyond – despite the impossibility of the task.

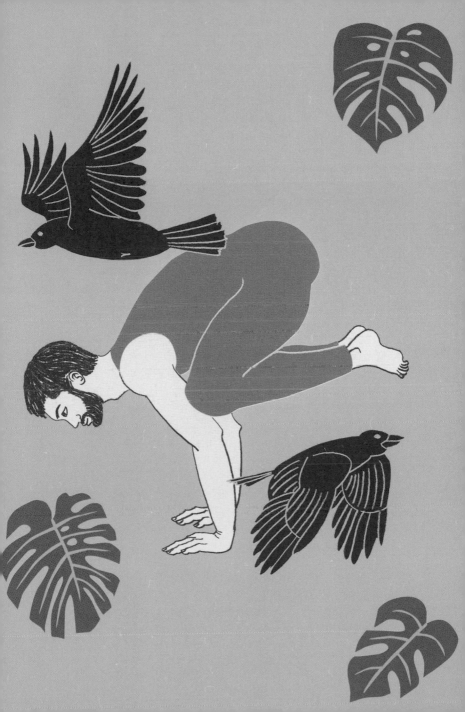

IN PRACTICE

Corvids in European culture are often portrayed as sinister as well as cunning. The magpie is a thief, the jackdaw a trickster, the raven a harbinger of death. But look closer and they reveal a real sense of fun. Google 'crow vs dog' if you'd like to lose half an hour watching mischievous corvids tweaking dogs' tails and playing ball. Or 'crows in snow' if you'd rather watch them sledding down roofs and making tiny snow angels. Although they share a basic anatomy, crows have none of the slightly pompous dignity of peacocks, or the watchful stillness of eagles. They quite like falling over and rolling on their backs.

Which is nice to bear in mind as you attempt to embody that avian defiance of gravity, folding your legs into wings and levering your body to perch on your bent forearms. When it comes to yoga *asana*, there are rising balances and sinking balances: in Tree pose, for example, the sense of weight travelling down into your roots gives a feeling of releasing downwards with gravity (*see also* p. 47). Crow is rather the opposite: an in-breath of a balance, defying gravity as you lift the weight up and away from the ground. Of course, Patanjali would have you keep the two in perfect balance, *sthira* and *sukha*. But remember, balance is not exactly the same as equilibrium. Crow must tend towards lightness and lift, even when underpinned by grounding and effort. Playful, jaunty and ready to topple over with good humour.

So, as you approach the conundrum of the Crow, it pays to spend longer than you might think gently rocking the weight between the balls of your feet and your hands. You're trying to soothe your mind and persuade it to unclench from a fierce concentration on the 'difficult' pose you're attempting to a looser, more playful engagement with the pose as a puzzle or game – a low-stakes enterprise. And don't forget, corvids use simple tools: try starting with a yoga block under your feet and positioning your mat facing the seat of a sofa or armchair, so that your forehead has somewhere safe to land.

HALF-MOON POSE
Ardha Chandrasana

....

WITH THE RIGHT LEG as support, pivot forwards 90 degrees from the hips, stretching your left leg straight out behind. Spreading both arms wide at shoulder height, rotate your torso and left leg 90 degrees to the left, so that your right fingertips point to the ground and your left fingertips to the sky. With a little imagination, you could draw a semi-circle from fingertip to fingertip, arcing around the outstretched leg, to make a flat half-moon.

IN CONTEXT

Our most intimate heavenly dancing partners, the sun and the moon, are locked into a syncopated rhythm with the Earth. A solar year – the time it takes the Earth to make one revolution around the sun – is 365 days long (give or take a few hours). A lunar year – the time it takes for the moon to orbit the Earth 12 times – is 11 days shorter, at 354 days. It's a calendar conundrum that different cultures have solved in different ways. The Gregorian calendar privileges the sun, adding additional days to the lunar months to bring the year up to quota – hence 'thirty days hath September, April, June ...' and so on. The Vedic calendar (in common with ancient Hebrew and Babylonian systems) is faithful to the 29-day-long lunar months, but adds a whole leap month every two to three years in order to stay in sync with the solar year. A complex set of calculations is required to ensure the appropriate festivals and rituals continue to match the agricultural seasons – keeping the sun and moon in balance is no trivial task.

The deity associated with the moon in Indian mythology is Chandra, a cool customer who earned renown by saving Shiva from

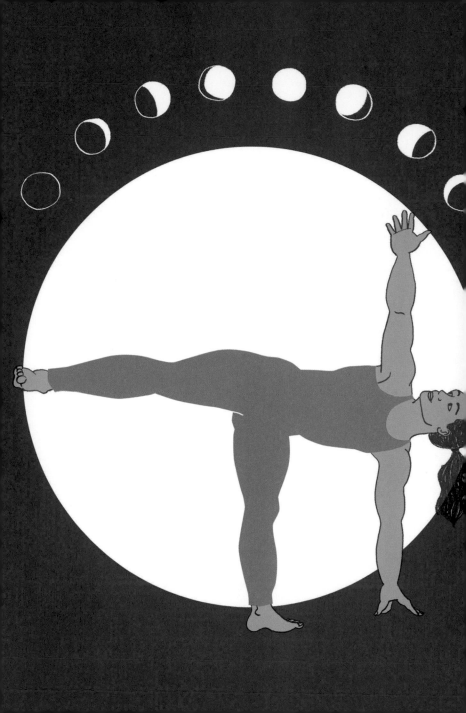

a deadly poison. He settled his pale orb on top of the god's head, and by virtue of his chilly nature drew out the 'heat' of the toxic fumes Shiva had inhaled. Of course, the moon represents the cool of night-time as a counterbalance to the day-time heat of the sun. The myth that explains his waxing and waning is a little less dignified.

The story goes that young Ganesh, the elephant-headed deity, was returning from a party one night, having overindulged in food and drink. He was more or less balanced on the back of his mouse, which was his usual steed, when a snake emerged and startled the little rodent. Ganesh toppled off and his belly split open, spilling out all the cakes and sweets he had eaten. With the resourcefulness of a true drunk, he simply stuffed them back in again, grabbed the snake and tied it around his middle to keep the food inside. Whereupon Chandra, who had been watching the antics, burst out laughing. In a fit of rage and injured dignity, Ganesh broke off one of his tusks and threw it at the moon, cursing him into darkness.

All was not well in the moonless world, however. Where previously Surya, the sun, and Chandra had taken turns to shine, now the land was baking under an endless day. Crops died, animals sickened and sleepless humans flipped back and forth between listlessness and rage. The gods summoned Ganesh and told him to fix the moon but no matter how hard he tried, the great Remover of Obstacles couldn't remove his own curse. The best he could do was to commute Chandra's sentence: from then on, the moon no longer shone full every night as he was used to. Instead his light gradually dimmed, then winked out, then slowly grew again, with just one day a month at its full strength. Even with these diminished powers, Chandra was able to re-establish the night-time and with it, the cooling darkness and sleep the world sorely needed.

One story about the origin of the word *hatha* suggests that its syllables signify sun (*ha*) and moon (*tha*). Scholars believe this association actually arose some time after hatha yoga got its name, but the explanation fits: hatha yoga contains plenty of sun and moon symbolism, thanks to the influence of tantric traditions.

The tantric body has two complementary energetic channels, or *nadi*: the left-hand one, called *ida*, is full of moon energy, while the sun moves in the right-hand channel, *pingala*. One of the yogin's key esoteric goals en route to liberation is to combine these sun and moon energies in such a way that a mysterious sacred energy called *kundalini* (which I'll discuss further in the Cobra pose, *see also* p. 125) can awaken and rise through a third, central channel (*sushumna nadi*) situated along the spine.

Through a metaphorical lens, we could say that the moon and sun represent the conjunction of opposites. We are being asked to enter into an alchemical process whereby day and night – like good and evil, or life and death – reveal themselves to be not binary opposites, but parts of a single interdependent whole. The fusion of these opposites unlocks tremendous power in the body of the adept.

IN PRACTICE

The precise process of folding and angling of the body into Halfmoon pose takes the sun-energy of flat geometric planes and the moon-energy of 3D spiral forms and merges them into a third thing that can feel a little uncanny, but strangely rewarding too.

It should go without saying that this one-legged, starfish-armed, hip-rotated pose is a challenge to your equilibrium. If your sense of balance tends to wax and wane – and it can be affected by tiredness, menstrual cycle, sinus congestion and stress, among other things – then start with your standing leg about 20 centimetres (8 inches) away from a wall and have a yoga block, or a stool or chair in front of you to rest your hand on.

Take your time and refuse to be flustered. Pay close attention to increasing your poise and control during the entry and exit phases as well as holding the pose. With practice, your pose can become a picture of cool and quiet: moonlight slanting in through a gap in the curtains and sliding across the wall.

LORD OF THE DANCE POSE
Natarajasana

....

STANDING ON ONE straight leg, crook the other leg back and lift it skywards to meet the same-side hand as it reaches behind to grasp the foot (and maybe even draws it up and over your head, if you are especially flexible). The other arm stretches gracefully in front for balance as your spine curves into a strong backbend.

IN CONTEXT

According to Hindu cosmology, the Earth and all it contains are not solid and stable, but rather the product of a rhythmic energetic vibration, a pattern of expansion and contraction played out across epochs called *yugas*. During a cycle lasting 4,320,000 years, four different *yugas* – ages of humankind – play out. The first, *satya yuga*, is the Age of Truth – similar to the ancient Greek concept of the Golden Age, a time of peace and plenty when Earth's bounty is freely given and shared by a noble race of humans. Each subsequent *yuga* sees the quality of life on Earth fall by a quarter: as wisdom and virtue decline, strife increases and even the climate becomes more hostile. The fourth age, *kali yuga*, sees the human race beset by darkness, ignorance and pollution. (You can probably guess which age we're in now.) As this final age comes to an end, the whole world is engulfed in flames so that it can begin again in a state of perfection with a new *satya yuga*.

The force that governs the whole process is the *tandava natyam*, the cosmic dance performed by Shiva in his guise as Nataraja, the Lord of the Dance. Whirling through phases of howling rage and ecstatic bliss, he dances the universe down the millennia to its fiery end, then dances it back into being all over again. As a symbol of cosmic energies, this dancing god has become something of a mascot to scientists with a mystical bent. There's a life-size sculpture of him in the courtyard of the European Organization for Nuclear Research (better known as CERN, home to the Large Hadron Collider). A gift from the Indian government, it bears a plaque with a quote from physicist and systems theorist Fritjof Capra reminding us that the 'metaphor of the cosmic dance unifies ancient mythology, religious art and modern physics'.

The CERN statue doesn't show Shiva in the yoga pose that bears his name – it turns out the Lord of the Dance has more than one shape to throw. The more common one in Hindu art and iconography is a different one-legged stance, both legs bent, the left leg and arm raised in front of him. Like the familiar yoga version illustrated here, that posture likely has its origins not in medieval hatha yoga but in Bharatanatyam, the oldest recorded form of Indian classical dance. *Natarajasana* is just one of around 20 poses found in modern yoga that appear to have their roots in this form of temple dance from Tamil Nadu in South India. Bharatanatyam is a form of physical culture that developed in parallel to hatha yoga, probably remaining largely separate until some of its shapes and gestures were borrowed by twentieth-century yoga modernisers in the neighbouring state of Mysore. It's significant to note that the Bharatanatyam tradition of dance performance belonged to women, whereas hatha yoga was primarily the preserve of men.

Modern global yoga, at least outside of India, has been such a female-dominated pursuit – surveys suggest that between 70 and 80 per cent of current practitioners are women – that we're inclined to look back at the history of hatha yoga with some dismay: where are all the women? Scholars believe there were some women who studied and performed yoga *asana* throughout its development,

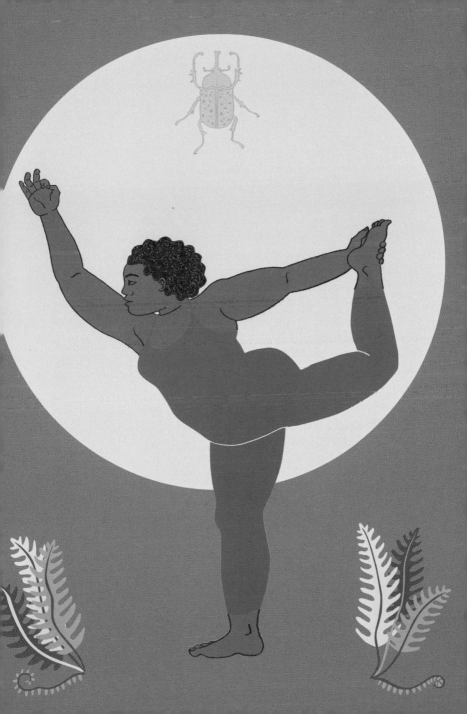

but they are next to invisible in the historical record before the twentieth century. At the same time, in our studies of yoga in the West we tend to overlook Indian classical dance completely – I don't remember it being mentioned in any of my course books during my teacher training. But surely these temple dancers and their fully developed language of expressive, graceful gestures must be an essential thread in the larger tapestry of yoga? In their performances we find smooth, flowing transitions from one gesture to the next; a group of women moving in unison; an emphasis on lightness, grace and balance: all familiar scenes at your local yoga studio today, but not apparent in the textual records of hatha yoga.

Given the affinities and exchanges between dance and yoga in India, it's no great surprise to find that here in the UK and in North America, yoga and contemporary dance have likewise been in profound and mostly fruitful conversation for more than a century. Many of the most influential female yoga teachers have come from a dance background and have recognised in the forms of postural yoga some lineaments of their former art. Blanche DeVries – probably the first American woman to make a career as a yoga teacher (and, incidentally, aunt to Theos Bernard, whose story we'll get to in the next chapter, *see also* p. 91) began as a proponent of 'Oriental Dance'. This system of harmonic gymnastics was a popular fitness craze in the early years of the twentieth century, despite having no authentic roots in any dance tradition of the 'Orient'. It brought a perfumed breeze of acceptable exoticism into the lives of middle-class American women and cross-pollinated freely with hatha yoga in the hands of DeVries and others. Indra Devi (born Eugenia Peterson), who repackaged hatha yoga for the same demographic in the 1950s, was an actor and dancer who briefly studied classical dance in India. Today, you'll find dance studies on the early resumés of plenty of influential teachers, including Sharon Gannon and Shiva Rea in the US and Angela Farmer, Catherine Annis and Tara Fraser in the UK.

IN PRACTICE

You don't have to be a trained ballerina to find the expressive grace of dance within the forms of yoga and *natarajasana* is a good place to start. Providing you are generally strong and flexible with no lower back issues, I'd be inclined to focus more on expression than alignment and really enjoy the swooping, *Swan Lake* drama of this backbend/balance combination. Have a sturdy chair nearby so that you can rest your leading hand on it, if necessary. If you have a good grip of your raised foot, concentrate on pressing it up and away into your hand to unlock a sense of lift and lightness in the pose.

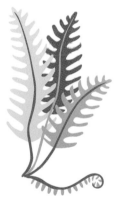

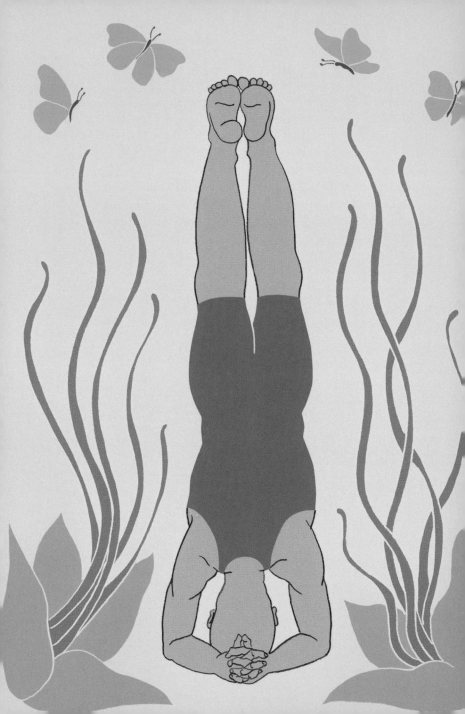

HEADSTAND
Sirsasana

....

*'Place the head on the ground and the feet up to the sky, for
a second only, and increase this time daily. After six months
wrinkles and grey hair are not seen. He who practises it daily,
even for three hours, conquers death.'*

HATHAYOGAPRADIPIKA III 81-82

IN CONTEXT

In the late summer of 1936, a young American graduate student
arrived in India, determined to learn the *real* yoga. Theos Bernard
was a social-climbing scholar from a colourful family: his uncle
Pierre was better known as 'Oom the Omnipotent', a tantric sex
guru who scandalised and hypnotised New York high society
during the Jazz Age. Newly married to psychoanalyst and heiress
Viola Wertheim, Theos finally had the funds he needed to pursue
his studies to their source.

Bernard embarked on a 'Grand Tour' of India's key cultural and
spiritual sites, eventually settling in the hills outside Ranchi as the
pupil of an esteemed teacher of traditional hatha yoga methods.
His studies began with a rigorous programme of yoga *asana*, to
prepare his body for the more strenuous purifications, breath work
and meditation that would follow. According to him, he always
finished his physical practice with a headstand – 'one of the most
important postures that I was required to perfect'.

'At first it seemed hopeless, especially when I found that the
standard for perfection is three hours.' Over the course of several

months of dedicated daily yoga practice, adding a minute a week, he built up to 15 minutes in the pose. By the end of the year, he claims to have achieved the three-hour goal. Conquering death proved harder; despite his extraordinary headstand prowess, Bernard was shot dead by Lahouli tribesmen 10 years later, during a field trip to the Punjab.

To understand the yogic significance of turning the body upside down, we need to lay down some basic tantric lore. Let's imagine that the body contains a sacred nectar, *amrita*, that is produced inside the head. Unless this nectar can somehow be dammed up at its source, it drips downwards from the palate and its life force is lost – either consumed by fire in the stomach or ejaculated as semen. There are a variety of yogic techniques aimed at keeping this nectar of immortality inside the practitioner's head. The most basic of these – like the headstand – use gravity. Simply turn the pot of the skull upside down and nothing can drip out.

These days, most yoga practitioners prefer a more prosaic explanation. It's fairly common to claim that the headstand rejuvenates the brain and vital organs by reversing the effects of gravity on the circulatory system and increasing blood flow to the brain. This is partially accurate: in fact, the body is so good at regulating blood pressure that the blood flow to the brain is increased only very slightly. The inversion strengthens venous return from the legs and torso, which does indeed increase blood flow to the heart. The resulting rise of pressure in the right atrium signals it to slow its rhythm. The strongest positive outcome of an inversion may be its effect on the nervous system: slower heartbeats induce a calming, 'rest and digest' response.

Whether it's due to the conservation of sacred nectar or the activation of the parasympathetic nervous system, there's no doubt that turning upside down can be strangely revitalising. I keep an expensive yoga toy in my office: a sleek, padded stool with a notch for my neck that lets me pop up into a headstand with my head floating safely six inches above the ground. I swear by it as a cure for writerly blockages and any situation where I've thought myself into a dead end. Turning my perspective upside down, just for 60 seconds, seems to shake something loose, to unjam my brain.

IN PRACTICE

I hate to be a bore, but the human shoulder girdle and cervical vertebrae were not designed to bear the whole weight of the body. There is nothing normal, natural or indeed necessary about standing on your head. The benefits of an inversion on the circulatory and nervous systems can be achieved by any pose that puts the hips above the heart – lying down with legs up the wall, for example. Meanwhile, the recorded risks from repeatedly trying to balance your bodyweight on the crown of your head include nerve damage such as thoracic outlet syndrome (compression of the nerves running from your neck to your arms), degenerative arthritis in the neck and retinal tears due to increased pressure on the eyes.

For me, the headstand belongs firmly in the category of intrinsically pointless things that people do just because they can – like juggling or learning Dothraki. There are safer and more accessible ways to get all the physical benefits of an inversion, so please practise the headstand purely for the joy of doing something difficult, for the change of perspective and the overcoming of a fear, not because of any dubious claims about its health benefits. And do so like Theos Bernard: slowly, diligently, guided by a teacher and in manageable increments.

Here's a thought experiment that you can do in any comfortable inversion: if you're an experienced yoga practitioner with no neck or shoulder issues, that might be a headstand. (And if you're a cheat like me, you can use a headstand stool.) Otherwise, it will work best to lie down with your buttocks close to a wall and your legs resting up the wall; prop your hips up on a bolster or a couple of folded blankets. Spend a few moments visualising the *amrita*, golden nectar of immortality, pooling in your head. Imagine the rejuvenating effects of conserving this life force. Take a rest in Child's pose (*see also* p. 141) or a similar introverted posture, if you need to.

Now take your inversion again, and this time visualise your physical circulatory system: the heart beating calmly and peacefully as blood flows effortlessly down from your feet to your chest. Notice the differences for you between activating a more esoteric, poetic narrative for your embodied experience versus a more anatomical, scientific one. Which feels more intriguing to you? Which is more comforting? What advantages and disadvantages does each perspective hold?

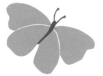

PEACOCK POSE
Mayurasana/Pincha Mayurasana

....

THE PEACOCK – or male Indian peafowl – is arguably the world's fanciest pheasant. Resplendent in iridescent royal blue and emerald green livery, with his cheeky feathered crown and that insanely opulent tail, it's no wonder the peacock has been a symbol of royalty and divinity not just in Indian culture, but around the world, by virtue of his export to Persia, Greece and beyond.

The yoga poses named after him are pretty showy, too. *Mayurasana* always reminds me of the short-lived 'planking' craze that broke the internet in 2011: the practitioner balances on the palms of his hands, arms bent at the elbow and elbows pressed together against his belly, plank-straight body and legs parallel to the floor. This echoes the shape of a peacock in repose, tail held daintily just above the dust. *Pincha mayurasana* – Peacock Tail Feather pose – is a forearm balance, with the body arching up away from the ground to mimic the erect tail feathers of the bird in full display.

IN CONTEXT

Peacock pose is the oldest non-seated yoga pose for which we have textual evidence. Written some time between the sixth and tenth century CE (Indian texts are notoriously difficult to date), the *Vimanarcanakalpa* gives the following instruction: 'Fix the palms of the hands on the floor, place the elbows on either side of the navel, raise the head and feet and remain in the air like a staff.' This is a big moment for hatha yoga, at least in written form. Any poses described in earlier texts are seated or kneeling positions that the practitioner is expected to hold for long periods, in the interests of meditation. With Peacock pose, a new element of balance with physical exertion is introduced.

The text goes on to dismiss the pose as one of the lowest, or least valuable – but nevertheless, it marks the moment when hatha yoga begins to embrace poses that are more visually striking and performative – Insta-worthy, in modern terms. Many of these early 'display' poses are named for birds and animals, and allow the yogin to channel the energies of the creatures they depict. For example, peacocks were widely supposed to eat poison in order to make themselves immune to it; likewise, Peacock pose was said to burn away the effects of bad food and stoke the digestive fires to better deal with toxins.

Later yoga texts enumerate at least six different types of Peacock pose, but none seems to be the inverted forearm balance beloved of twenty-first-century yoga influencers. (If you do *pincha mayurasana* and nobody takes a photo, did it even happen?) There's no doubt it looks impressive, and it's fittingly named for a bird that's all about display. You may think I sound a bit dismissive – if so, you caught me. Those of us who like to think our approach to yoga is centred around inner experience and self-exploration, or the transcendence of the ego, can get sniffy about the show-off aspects of *asana* practice. It's an uncomfortable thing to explain away, and sometimes we protest too much. *I'm* not perfecting my body to impress others, the story goes. These lithe, strong limbs are an outward expression of discipline, *tapas*, and some kind of purity of soul. I am striking the pose of an authentic truth-seeker, but that influencer over there is just in it for the likes.

Perhaps this story we tell ourselves is sometimes true, at least for a given value of truth. But the idea that the outer form of the *asana* didn't matter at all until capitalism and social media corrupted yoga's inherent purity is lacking in nuance. As I mentioned in the

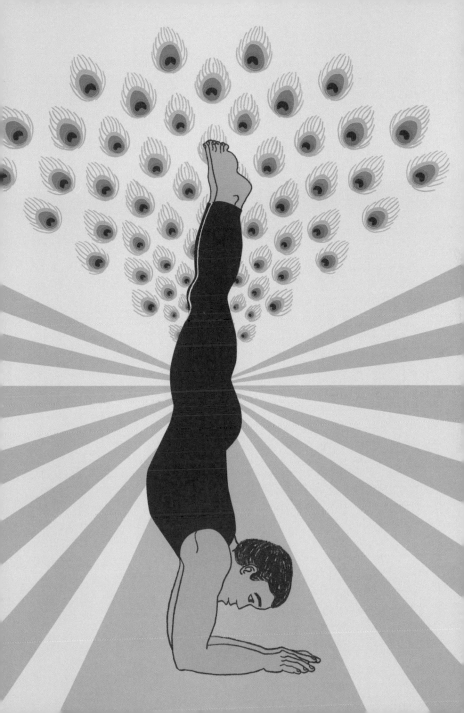

Sun Salutation section (*see also* p. 36), yoga's conundrum around monetisation didn't begin with branded yoga mats and overpriced activewear. From *sadhus* performing austerities in the marketplace in expectation of alms, to Krishnamacharya exhibiting his hyper-flexible pupils as a display of proud and potent young Indian manhood, to the present-day yoga teacher dependent on her Instagram following: the temptation to provide the crowd with yoga eye-candy has always been there. And so too have the disapproving critics, who dismiss it all as so much acrobatics.

IN PRACTICE

One reason these postures are so eye-catching is that a body balanced in such an unusual orientation looks deeply odd, like a three-dimensional optical illusion. To mimic the lightness and grace of a peacock, in poses that require significant exertion and precise balance, is not easy or natural. A strong core and upper body and flexible but well-supported shoulder joints are prerequisites. (As a cautionary note, take care not to strain the wrists in basic Peacock and the shoulders and neck in Tail Feather pose.) A lighter body type helps, too. But the distribution of body weight in space is the real key.

The would-be peacock must pay close moment-by-moment attention to their centre of gravity and position in space, while making the cognitive adjustments for being prone (face down), or upside down. You'd better hope that the concentration required to do this safely is enough to take your focus off the performance aspect; I can tell you from painful experience that showing off to a spectator is the number-one yoga activity most likely to result in injury. One way to shift your mindset away from performance is to really immerse yourself in the journey. These are poses you need to work towards and train for, and that's the point – much more than the final display.

5
TWISTING

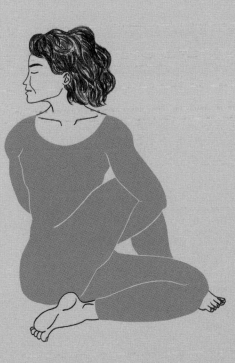

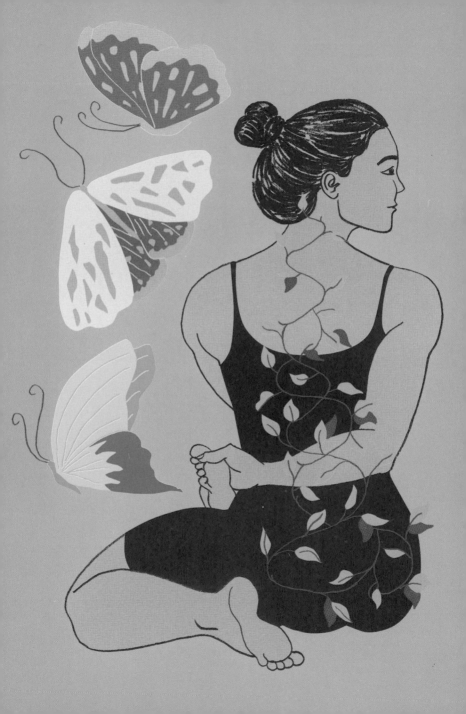

BHARADVAJA'S POSE
Bharadvajasana

....

SOMETIMES MY CAT ends up in an awkward position; the urge to climb up all of the things will get you that way. Perched on top of a fence post, trying to fit all four paws on to a two-by-four square, she's not exactly relaxed – and yet there's something poised and graceful about her, always. It's the same energy I see in the pose belonging to the sage Bharadvaja.

To make this off-kilter kneeling shape, you need to shift your hips so they sit to one side of your shins and twist your torso away from your legs. Once settled, turn your face to look back towards your feet for a distinctly feline vibe. It's awkward and elegant at once.

IN CONTEXT

Bharadvaja, so the story goes, was a dedicated student of the Vedas. He spent three lifetimes memorising scriptures, practising austerities and denying himself the society of other people in the hope that his devotions would move the gods to liberate him from the cycle of death and rebirth. As he lay dying for the third time, chanting mantras in his lonely cell, the god Shiva appeared at his bedside. Bharadvaja stirred and whispered, 'At last! Are you going to take me away?' Shiva shook his head. 'What good is all this learning when you never shared it? Each lifetime, you plucked a mere handful of dust from a mountain of knowledge. You have nothing to show for it.'

Bharadvaja wept silently. Shiva was moved to pity and told him, 'You have one more chance. If, during your next lifetime, you use your learning to uplift others, then I will release you.' Thus rebooted, Bharadvaja spent a long life as a teacher, touching the lives of thousands of people. On his deathbed for a fourth time, he found himself surrounded by loving students. As he slipped away, Shiva appeared to him once more and opened his arms. 'Welcome! Consider your life's work done. Are you ready to come home?' But Bharadvaja shook his head: 'Let me do it again, Lord!' And he reincarnated as a great sage to share his wisdom with the world all over again.

The symbolism of Bharadvaja's story is played out in the contradictions of his pose. He twists his spine first one way, then his gaze back the other way: drawn towards the divine, but also back to the world. He is poised but awkward, giving up the prize of liberation in order to stay human and fallible.

I'll tell you a secret – although if you're a yoga teacher, you should already know it: most yoga teachers are not innately stronger or more perfect than their students. Most of us are wounded people who have found a medicine that works for us and want to share it with the world. This can make us incredibly empathetic and effective. It can also blind us to the different needs, the different wounds our students may be carrying. Greek mythology gives us the myth of Chiron, a centaur who served as a great teacher to all the heroes and was credited with inventing the arts of healing – both herbal medicine and surgery. Struck by accident with a poisoned arrow, he suffered such chronic pain that he eventually renounced his immortality rather than live any longer. He gives us the archetype of the 'wounded healer': teachers who can help everyone except themselves and whose wounds eventually make it impossible for them to continue teaching.

Bharadvaja offers a different and more hopeful paradigm of teaching: as an escape from solipsism, a route out of the self through sharing time and knowledge with others. But for me he also embodies the contradictory stance of the yoga teacher, who is never far from that inner tug-of-war between their own self-practice and development and the needs of their students. And although Bharadvaja never had to curate his personal brand on social media, I bet he experienced the discomforts of having his lifestyle held up as an exemplar to his students; the pressure to either hide his wounds or turn them into an improving narrative full of teachable moments. Yoga teachers today still find themselves walking this line.

IN PRACTICE

Negotiating those contradictory forces can make a person pretty anxious, and likewise this pose can take on a sort of coiled spring vibe. But I think it's really about finding peace with the contradictions, and accepting that the path we take is always winding. There is a gorgeous photo, reproduced in the introduction to T.K.V. Desikachar's book *The Heart of Yoga*, that purports to show the Maharaja of Kolhapur demonstrating *Bharadvajasana* in 1940. Now, this is definitely not true, because the Associated Press reported the death of that same royal gentleman from a heart attack in November of that year, at the age of 43, and noted in passing that he weighed 280 pounds (127 kilos). So the identity of the slender young man in the photograph remains a mystery (perhaps he was the Maharaja's yoga teacher?) but his poise and charisma are beyond doubt. He wears tiny white shorts, the better for us to appreciate the clean lines of his torso and jawline – oh, and his flawless execution of the pose. His left foot is hooked into the crook of his right thigh in a half-Lotus position and his left arm reaches around to 'bind' with the left foot, unquestionably the most demanding expression of this pose. Yet his face, tilted ever so slightly to look over his right shoulder, is both keenly alert and utterly serene.

I could tell you to approach this pose with the patience of a three-lifetime sage and the ease of a sunflower turning its face to follow the day. You could tell me to sod off. But actually, the image that helps me most is that of a climbing plant. Think of your spine as a pliant stalk, and let it unfurl upwards from the tipped pot of your pelvis in what feels like quite a natural, soft spiral. Resist the urge to prop or lever with the arms. When the twist is very well and easefully established, turn your gaze back past your other shoulder into the soft middle distance, and let the weight of your head follow.

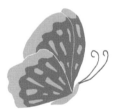

MATSYENDRA'S POSE
Matsyendrasana

....

IT'S A GOOD THING this book is illustrated, because some yoga poses defy verbal description. Still, here goes: from a seated position, bend both knees and tuck your right foot under your left leg to lie alongside the left hip, so that the outer side of your right leg is resting on the ground. Step the left foot over your bent right knee, so that the sole of your foot is flat on the floor next to the right thigh, with the left knee pointing up to the ceiling. Now twist your spine towards the upward-pointing left knee, resting your left hand on the ground behind you and tucking the outer elbow of your right arm against the outer edge of the left knee. To achieve the fullest expression of the pose, reach your left hand further around behind your back and bend your right arm at the elbow, turning at the shoulder to reach back and clasp your hands behind you. Got that? Good, now do the other side.

IN CONTEXT

This double-angled spinal twist is named for Matsyendra, which means Lord of the Fishes. His origin story is one of those myths that lends itself to narrative embroidery: there are a number of different versions, each more colourful than the last. My favourite is the one that begins with a baby boy born under an inauspicious star. Warned by an astrologer that their son will be very unlucky, his parents throw their baby into the nearest river. At once, the child is swallowed up by a great big fish, thereby neatly fulfilling the astrologer's prophecy.

By rights, that should be the end of the story – but there's a twist in this fishy tale. Somehow, the child grows up to be a wise, curious and well-adjusted boy, despite spending the first 12 years of his life inside an actual fish. One day he hears the voice of the god Shiva, who is sitting on the riverbank, teaching his wife Parvati the secrets of yoga. Intrigued by what he hears and curious to learn more, he speaks to the god from inside the fish. Shiva is moved to rescue him. Perhaps because of his unorthodox upbringing, once released he turns out to be not quite human, but rather a sort of merman: part person, part fish. Under Shiva's instruction, Matsyendra (for it is he) goes on to become a great yoga teacher himself, and the teachings he passes on to his descendant Swatmarama are eventually recorded in the fifteenth-century yoga manual known as the *Hathayogapradipika*.

This story makes a nice pair with the one I'll tell later on (*see also* Cobra, p. 123), about the great sage Patanjali being half man, half water snake, found in a river. It means that both Patanjali's Yoga Sutras and Swatmarama's *Hathayogapradipika* – two of the foundational texts of modern yoga – are attributable to chimeric beings who are part human, part lithe, slithery water-creature.

There's a liminal flavour to these origin stories that situates yoga itself as a creature of the riverbank, making its home in between the solid ground of worldly concerns and the shimmering waters of the esoteric realm. It also reflects hatha yoga's history as a fringe religious practice: the preserve of people who choose to set themselves apart from the normies. The semi-mythical sage Matsyendra is identified as one of the founders of the Nath Order of yogins: ash-smeared, forest-dwelling tantric adepts who are credited with the invention of hatha yoga in the Middle Ages. Hailing from the lower rungs of the social ladder, these yogins renounced the solid ground of the established social order to splash in the deep waters of tantric ritual, which included breaking

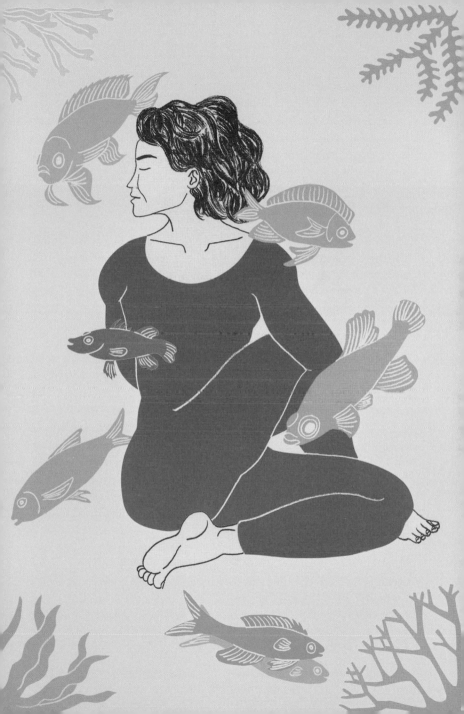

taboos around 'unclean' foods, alcohol and sex.

And perhaps Matsyendra's story also contains an allusion to the fluid flexibility of the fish's spine. The yogin in *asana* must transcend the limitations of his human frame and become something at once more creaturely and more magical. You need to tap into a certain amphibious quality in order to fold your body into the pose of Matsyendra, a mer-boy tucked inside a fish's belly.

IN PRACTICE

Matsyendra's pose tests the flexibility of hips, shoulders and spine, but the biggest challenge in this pose might be to maintain a full, steady breath: the compression of the spinal twist against the thigh can make you wish you had gills to supplement the meagre space available for your lungs. To facilitate better breathing, you need good structure and an unpushy attitude. For structure, ensure that the sitting bones are well balanced and grounded – you may need to modify your leg position to allow this. From this stable base, let the spine be very upright – propping the sitting bones on a block or folded blanket should help.

Now, before you begin the twist, check in with yourself. Are you focused on a goal, perhaps to bind or reach a certain degree of rotation? Drop it. Instead, let your belly be very soft and liquid. I like to imagine I'm a bag of water with a goldfish inside and the fish is swimming around in the direction I want to rotate. If you get stuck, untwist a tiny bit and wait – a few beats longer than you want to. Now let your eyes travel just ahead of you and see if your spine wants to follow them on into the twist.

Let the journey be endless and the goal irrelevant: you're looking for a fishy sort of drift where your ribs flex like gills and you can float on the currents of your breath. As soon as you find yourself fixating on an end point, the fluidity and softness of the swimming fish will vanish and you'll find yourself back on land, ratcheting your elbow against your knee and holding your breath.

MARICHI'S POSE
Marichyasana

....

Marichyasana is, at its heart, a seated pose with one leg extended along the ground and the other one bent. Around this foundation, a series of four variations takes shape. For starters, there's a bound forward bend and a bound twist (meaning the arms are wrapped in a loop around the bent leg and the body, the hands clasped to 'bind' the pose in place). For extra experience points, these can also be practised with the extended leg bent and the foot tucked into the crook of the opposite thigh (sometimes called a 'half-Lotus'), giving two more variations. These more extreme expressions of the pose resemble human knots: the contortions of a magician's assistant whose job is to hide inside a suitcase.

IN CONTEXT

The series of seated poses named for the sage Marichi is not recorded before the twentieth century, when it was described and named by Krishnamacharya and went on to become a key part of the primary series of his student Pattabhi Jois's ashtanga vinyasa yoga method. But the myth of Marichi is much older. In Hindu mythology he is one of the Manasaputras, the seven sons born from the mind of Brahma the divine creator. He is the grandfather of the sun god Surya and the great-grandfather of Manu, the father of humanity.

Although one of the Sanskrit meanings of *marichi* is 'ray of light', the stories about him have more of a 'malevolent narcissist' vibe. When he wasn't helping to create the universe, Marichi lived with his wife Dharmavrata. One day he returned home extremely tired and told her to wash his feet. This chore was interrupted by

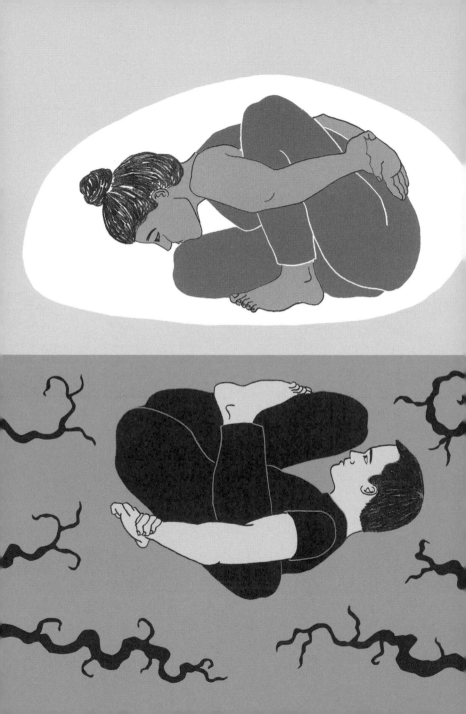

the arrival of his father, Brahma, whereupon Dharmavrata stopped washing her husband's feet in order to welcome their divine guest. Marichi was so enraged by this slight to his status that he immediately put a curse on his wife that turned her to stone.

After many years spent in patient meditation – after all, what else could she do in her mineralised state? – Dharmavrata caught the attention of Lord Vishnu (one of the principal Hindu deities). He took pity on her and offered her a favour. When she replied that she would actually quite like not to be a rock, he shook his head sadly. 'Your husband's curse is too strong,' he told her. 'But I can make you into a really cool sort of rock, with holy powers, that all the gods will want to own.' So he did. Afterwards Dharmavrata was still a rock, but a rock that men fought over, and now she had the rest of eternity to figure out why that was supposed to be better.

It's not clear to me whether the people who attached his name to these postures approved of Marichi's approach to marital disputes, but having learned his story it's hard not to see something of the furious, clenched character of the vengeful husband in these knotted twists and binds. Or shades of the petrified wife, folded into a suitcase of stone, forever. Which raises the question: if these ancient, fearful tales are written into the poses, do we become complicit when we practise them? And is it possible – or right or useful – to somehow rewrite the stories? To exorcise the violent ghosts that inhabit these shapes and find new metaphors?

On such matters, I have reached a place of tentative resolution. I refuse to ignore or overwrite stories just because they are 'Not Nice'. I'm not interested in changing the name of the pose, or finding a more hopeful reading of the myth. But on the other hand, I don't want to leave Marichi's status and deeds unquestioned. So it becomes a question of finding a way to practise the poses in awareness of the story of Dharmavrata and Marichi, with all its pitiless fatalism. Here is the monstrous fragility of a male ego; here is the violence projected out into the world; here is the woman silenced with no recourse to justice. Here is one of the oldest human knots, and the hardest to untie. But at the same time, look: here is my agency in doing this practice, in this way, in this time and place. And after a while, I break free of the pose – because I am not turned to stone, and never will be.

IN PRACTICE

In the ashtanga primary series, the forward bending variations of Marichi's pose come first, followed by the twists. The theory is that a forward bend creates length and space in the spine, which facilitates a freer twist afterwards. You'll want to be quite warm and limber to begin with – these poses come about an hour into the series, after a whole lot of dynamic movement and stretching.

Heroic attempts to 'go for the bind' before your shoulders are ready will come back to bite you (make sure your teacher knows this too, especially if they are keen on hand-on adjustments). It's much better to concentrate on a nice, free line in the spine first, with the aim that the eventual clasping of the hands will happen without strain. An important caveat, seldom discussed in yoga classes: binding is a function of lean bodies, long limbs and a natural tendency towards flexibility. This last condition starts with individual physiology; although yoga can help us limber up, it can't change the basic structure of our joints. For those of us who carry more mass, inhabit a more compact frame, or are not born bendy, the laws of physics may prevent our arms from ever encircling the leg and the body at once.

Marichyasana, like its namesake sage, is an uncompromising pose. But that doesn't mean we shouldn't find ways to soften it. A bit of lift under the hips is useful – a thin block or folded blanket facilitates the forward bend and supports the twist. And why not use a strap to 'cheat' the bind, by grasping it in both your hands to span any gap between them? Call it a small act of resistance: showing compassion to the angry Marichi and his poor stony wife by making them both a bit more comfortable.

6
BENDING

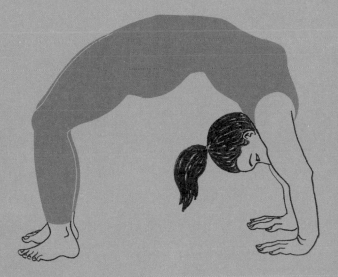

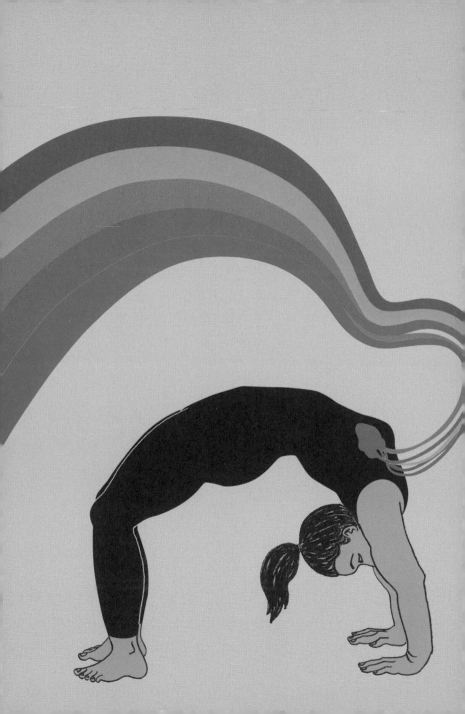

UPWARD-FACING BOW POSE
Urdhva Dhanurasana

....

HERE IS THE QUINTESSENTIAL backbend: hands and feet plant themselves flat on the ground, while the whole front side of the body arcs up to the sky like a rainbow. It's what we used to call 'The Crab' in school gymnastics class, as we went scuttling around, taking our youthful flexibility for granted. Older adults may relate more to the metaphor of a bridge, bolted together from rusty girders and creaking in the wind. Whatever your baseline level of bendiness, it's a powerful pose with some profound mood-altering capabilities.

IN CONTEXT

I wonder how much you can tell about a culture from the stories it tells about the rainbow. In Hindu mythology, it's Indra's bow: the weapon of the god of thunder and war, who uses it to shoot arrows of lightning. In Greek and Norse myths, it's a divine highway or bridge across the sky. In Aboriginal folklore, it's a colourful serpent. In Ireland, where my own ancestors originate, it's a confidence trick with a pot of fool's gold at the end.

Not everyone trusts a rainbow. It's a bit too shiny, too good to be true. But it's also glorious: spirit-lifting in its beauty, a brief shout of defiance against the rain and the darkness. Strong backbends like this one have definite rainbow energy. They can induce something like euphoria – just check out the glowing, borderlineculty faces of the students floating out of a backbend-heavy yoga workshop, some of them tear-stained with the after-effects of all the emotional release. In the parlance of yogaland, backbends 'open the heart' and 'release negative emotions stored in the body'. An awful lot of studio classes during the commercial yoga boom of the last two decades have traded on this language, combined with the highs of the physical practice of back bending. It feels cathartic to crack open your heart chakra and let everything out.

The shiny, happy yogins aren't making it up: the feel-good effects of facing life with a broad, open chest can also be observed in laboratory conditions. There's a strong association between posture, mood and mental attitude. To pick just one of many similar studies, a 2014 randomised controlled trial assigned participants either an upright or a slumped posture while they completed various tasks and conversations. The upright group reported 'higher self-esteem, more arousal, better mood, and lower fear' compared to their hunched counterparts, who used 'more negative emotion words, [...] sadness words, and fewer positive emotion words and total words' during the exercises – suggesting that even a slight extension of the spine can lift your mood. Another study 'dosed' depressed patients with yoga and found that their MRI scans revealed elevated levels of a chemical called GABA for approximately four days after each class. Gamma-aminobutyric acid is an amino acid that acts as a neurotransmitter in the central nervous system and has been associated with decreased depressive symptoms.

From a purely physical point of view, back bending has profound benefits too. Spinal extension (the technical term for bending the spine backwards) stretches the tissues on the front side of the body. One of the structures that benefits from this action is the diaphragm: the unique dome-shaped muscle that sits in between the lungs and the abdominal organs, and which is key to the action of breathing. As you breathe in, the diaphragm tightens and flattens to create a vacuum that sucks air into the lungs – imagine putting up an umbrella by pulling the handle down while you hold on to the ring that connects the spokes, and you have a decent working schematic of the diaphragm and its central tendon. As you breathe out, the central tendon/umbrella handle releases the softening diaphragm back up into the chest cavity. A tight, weak diaphragm means shallow, ineffective breathing. A strong, supple one ... you get the picture. Regular back bending – it doesn't have to be extreme at all – helps to keep the diaphragm in shape, with the result that normal breathing becomes more efficient and less effortful.

Stretching the spine often means stretching an artery, too. In a backbend, the body's main artery – the aorta – and the crucial femoral arteries that supply your legs are also subject to gentle extension. Studies have confirmed that people with more flexible spines have less arterial stiffness. Arterial stiffening is associated with increased risk of conditions like high blood pressure, diabetes and even organ failure. The flexibility of the arterial walls naturally declines as we age, but regular gentle stretching can go a long way to help maintain healthy arteries.

For me, this is a nice example of how science and metaphor can sit side by side, two parallel languages to illuminate the same experience. Knowing that your GABA levels are elevated after a yoga class doesn't wholly explain the way you feel, just as describing the opening of your heart doesn't do full justice to the intricate systems that govern your arterial flexibility.

IN PRACTICE

Now, without mentioning leprechauns, let me just remind you of the rainbow's illusory and temporary nature. Just like that pretty sliver of refracted sunshine, the backbend high is not sticking around forever. On a residential yoga retreat, a good teacher will put 'peak backbend day' in the middle, so that everyone has space and time to deal with the emotional catharsis and the ensuing comedown. In a regular class, you want plenty of time afterwards to cool down with gentle forward bends and so on. There is absolutely nothing wrong with using backbends to lift your mood; I would just invite you to notice what's happening, and strive for balance.

Talking about the Upward-facing Bow pose as a heart opener distracts from the fact that it's an equal challenge for the front of the hips and thighs. The back can't bend if the front can't open: preparatory poses should pay attention to the whole front line of the body, particularly from knees to nose. When opening up into the full expression of the pose, think length and space: the knees and elbows moving away from one another to create lots of room for your spine to curve upwards.

In the end, it's worth keeping in mind that there are many kinds of bridges, from a log laid across a stream, to the Golden Gate, to the Bifrost rainbow bridge to Asgard in Norse mythology: all have their rightful function. Similarly, all intensities of backbend have potential benefits for your body and mind – you get to decide whether today is a log day, or a Bifrost day.

BOW POSE
Dhanurasana

....

CONSIDER THE PHYSICS of the bow: as the archer applies tension to the centre of the bowstring, force is exerted evenly on the two extremes of the bow and its curve irresistibly deepens. In its tensioned shape, the bow stores the strength of the archer, waiting to transfer all of it into the arrow's swift forward motion. To assume the pose that bears its name, you must start on your belly on the ground, knees bent and arms reaching back to grasp the ankles. Your body from knees to shoulders represents the rigid part of the bow; the lower legs and the arms represent the bowstring. Now imagine an invisible archer, taking hold of your 'string' and drawing it upwards to bend your body into an elegant, springy curve. Your balance point – the centre of your curved frontage – is the spot where the arrow would take aim, firing straight down into the earth.

IN CONTEXT

The mythical prince Arjuna, hero of the *Bhagavad Gita*, was a legendary archer. One story illustrates his prowess with bow and arrow. Arjuna and his brothers had a teacher named Drona and one day, he gathered all the princes for a test of their skill. After placing a model bird high in the branches of a tree, he called the boys one by one to step forwards and shoot the bird's eye. First up was Yudhisthira; once he had drawn his bow, Drona asked him, 'What do you see?' 'The bird, the tree, my brothers and my bow in my hand,' he replied. Drona told him to stand down and called up the next pupil, then the next – but all gave the same answer. Finally, he called Arjuna forwards and asked him, 'What do you see?'

Arjuna replied, 'I see the bird's eye. That is all.' His teacher instructed him to shoot, and Arjuna's arrow flew straight and true through the centre of the eye.

In this account, Arjuna's bow acts like a magical lens, focusing his attention so perfectly on its target that there is nothing else in the world except the bird's eye: no tree, no brothers, no arrow – and no Arjuna. The bow is an instrument of self-dissolution, breaking down the distinctions between self, tool and purpose. It's a useful metaphor for yoga: a tool of enquiry that eventually collapses into its goal. In other words, we practise the techniques of yoga until we attain the state of yoga.

Compared to English, with its vast and precise vocabulary ideally suited to differentiating and labelling, the Sanskrit language is altogether more cryptic and allusive. It consists of a relatively small number of root words that can be modulated in various ways to create an almost infinite array of meanings. The same arrangement of letters can signify many things and whole philosophies can be – and have been – built on the ambiguities that ensue. For example, here's a far from exhaustive list of some of the meanings of the word 'yoga': a way or method; mixing or putting in order; a trick; an opportunity, undertaking or endeavour; gain or profit; diligence; magic; the act of fixing an arrow on the bow string; joining together, attaching or harnessing (the root word 'yuj' gives us the English 'yoke'). Depending on which source you're looking at, the sort of yoga we're dealing with in this book is sometimes a method – a system or set of techniques to harness the mind and body and orient them towards the goal of spiritual liberation – and sometimes the goal itself – an end-state of spiritual liberation. Yoga is the way, the means, and the end: the arrow, the bow, and the target.

IN PRACTICE

While you're *being* the bow, your nervous system is dealing with five or six distinct and novel physical challenges, including a deep bend in

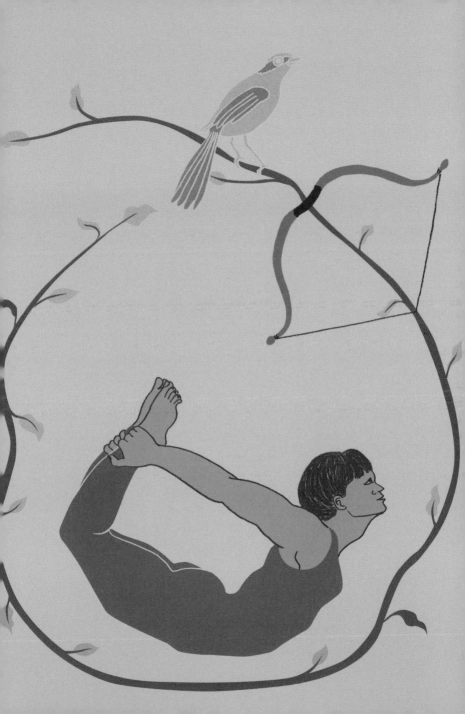

the lower back, full extension through the front of the hips, a strong sensation of opening across the chest, substantial unaccustomed force through the bent knees, and the challenge of breathing and balancing while experiencing all of the above. You're also working against gravity as you attempt to lift all the heaviest parts of the body – head, shoulders, hips, legs – up and away from the ground.

In the circumstances, it's quite hard to feel philosophical. But the difficulty is kind of the point. It's the reason why Zen Buddhists regard archery as a powerful form of meditative practice in its own right. Mustering the simultaneous strength and delicacy required to draw a heavy bow while also keeping your aim true, you become fully occupied – to the point of total absorption. You do all that heavy lifting to arrive at a state of lightness. At least, that's the idea. The beginning yoga student may soon become painfully aware that the Bow pose cannot be achieved by effort alone. Like the wood of the bow and the gut of the string, each part of the body needs to achieve the proper balance of give and resistance, elasticity and tension. It can help to think about the concept of the bow storing the strength of the archer in its taut string: imagine that the effort you put into the pose is being contained, rather than spent.

If you ever get a chance to try out an aerial yoga sling, especially with an experienced instructor, you'll get the delicious experience of making the bow shape while gravity works with, rather than against you. But short of finding a way to cheat gravity, there are some modifications you can try to make the pose feel less earthbound. First, prepare with plenty of warm-up poses that lengthen the fronts of the thighs and some that give you a gentle opening across the upper chest (these could include lunges, bridges and seated twists). Second, you could grab some props to play with. One option is a yoga belt or strong scarf to loop around your ankles, effectively giving you longer arms. Another is to prop your hips against a bolster so that it supports across the front of your pelvis and the top part of the pubic bone. Bending your knees and bringing heels towards buttocks, reach back with one hand at a time to take hold of your feet.

COBRA POSE
Bhujangasana

....

FROM A PRONE (face down) position on the floor, snake your chest up and out like a cobra's hood. Keep your hips resting on the ground and use your arms to prop yourself in place.

IN CONTEXT

India is home to almost 300 native snake species, of which about sixty are venomous. More than half of the world's snakebite deaths occur in India – over 50,000 a year on average – and the Indian cobra is one of the 'Big Four' deadliest species. With its distinctive hood and menacing upright fighting stance, the cobra is instantly recognisable – and instantly terrifying too. In fact, research suggests the human nervous system is hard-wired to respond to snake-shaped objects: experiments have repeatedly shown that both adults and young children visually detect snakes faster than any other kinds of stimuli – even when they have never seen one before.

With so many deadly snakes lurking around the place, it would be reasonable to expect them to be universally feared and vilified in Indian culture. Take the ancient Indian board game known as Mokshapat, the original Snakes and Ladders. Traditionally featuring just five ladders (faith, generosity, reliability, knowledge and our old friend *tapas*, *see also* p. 47) and a whopping 12 writhing snakes (including vulgarity, rage, drunkenness and murder), it's a great way to introduce your kids to the idea that they're only a dice-throw away from disaster. Teaching children to scale the ladders of virtue and avoid the snakes of evil feels like a familiar piece

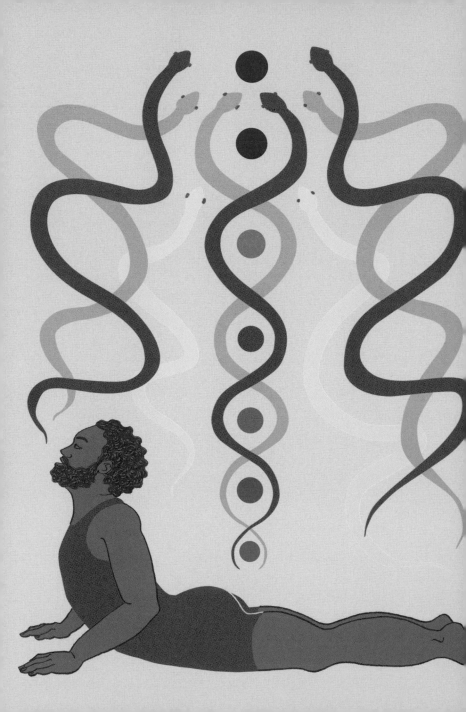

of Sunday School moral education. But unlike Judaeo-Christian mythology, in which the serpent is a guise for Satan and therefore the embodiment of evil, Indian spiritual traditions are much more sophisticated in their understanding of the snake's power and symbolism. It's an avatar of death, but also of reincarnation or immortality: the snake sheds its skin and is reborn anew, just as humans can shed their earthly bodies to inhabit their true nature as *brahman*, made of divine stuff. And it's also the symbol of the ultimate yoga secret sauce: *kundalini* energy.

Hatha yoga began as a synthesis of two older systems of energy management: from the ascetic tradition it took the notion of *tapas* and the idea of heating or burning impurities out of the body, while from the tantric tradition it adopted the idea of alchemical energetic processes that dissolve grosser elements into subtler ones. Tantra teaches that there are two types of energy: *prana*, or lifeforce, and *kundalini*, the mysterious serpent power. *Prana* is circulating at all times in a living body, and can be mastered and controlled by the techniques of *asana* (postural work) and *pranayama* (breath control). *Kundalini* is, for the majority of the time, asleep: she lies (she's definitely a feminine force, sometime described as a goddess) coiled three and a half times around the spot at the base of the spine called *muladhara chakra*. In twentieth-century Indologist and yoga scholar Georg Feuerstein's inimitably Teutonic phrase, this root chakra is 'the normally closed plug-hole to the infinite storehouse of Energy and Consciousness'.

Adepts who wish to open the plug-hole and awaken the Serpent Power are aiming for a sort of personal Big Bang, where the waves of *prana* meet the particles of *kundalini* and everything goes a bit quantum. They are advised to prepare to die: the *Gheranda Samhita* tells the yogin to smear himself in ashes. Through forceful breath retention exercises, some of which border on auto-asphyxiation, he must seize the serpent by her tail so that she rises up through the central channel of the spine, creating intense heat and vibrations, purifying and transmuting the bodily elements as she goes. Once *kundalini* reaches the crown chakra, the yogin gains enlightenment in the form of awareness of the oneness of all things.

It may sound pretty fantastical, but you can find multiple first-person accounts of this 'kundalini experience' in the modern era, both positive and negative. The practices prescribed for the awakening of *kundalini* can feel transformative; they can also bring on a spiritual emergency that is hard to distinguish from psychosis – the serpent is not to be trifled with.

Keeping your cool in the presence of poisonous snakes is a bit of a staple in Hindu iconography. The god Krishna is shown trampling the fearsome many-headed serpent Kaliya, while playing his flute with divine insouciance. The goddess Durga is usually depicted either subduing a snake with her foot or brandishing it in one of her 10 arms. Elephant-headed Ganesha wears one as a belt. Perhaps most impressively, Lord Vishnu sleeps peacefully on the hood of a giant cobra named Shesha.

One of the quirkiest serpent myths of all is the one that claims the sage Patanjali, credited with the authorship of the Yoga Sutras, was half man, half water snake. The story goes that Vishnu's aforementioned serpent sidekick Shesha, whose broad and comfy back served as the god's mattress, got interested in yoga. So his master promised he would be incarnated as a great yogi. Cut to a riverbank, where a yogini (a semi-divine female yoga adept) named Gonika was sitting in meditation. She prayed to the gods to send her a son to whom she could pass on all her knowledge. When her practice was done, she scooped up some water in her cupped hands and – to her shock and amazement – saw that she had picked up a tiny snake with a boy's head. (Or possibly a child with a snake's tail. Or a snake that turned into a boy. Eyewitness accounts vary.) He asked her to teach him all she knew, and she named him Patanjali, from *pata*, fallen, and *anjali*, the name for hands folded in prayer. Like the origin myth of Matsyendra, the Lord of the Fishes, I like to think that this story gifts one of the founding fathers of yoga with an enviably sinuous, snaky spine – ideal for poses like Cobra.

IN PRACTICE

I'm going to suggest two seemingly contradictory considerations for this pose. (In case it's not clear by now, that's very much the yogic way of things.)

First, remember that snakes don't have arms. The sense of lift and strength in this pose should come from the torso, as the back muscles lift and support and the front line lengthens and softens.

Second, pay close attention to your arms: you're going to have to put them somewhere, because you are not actually a snake. Placement of the hands should be very deliberate, and entirely idiosyncratic. Start with your hands wherever they need to be in order to keep your shoulders relaxed away from your ears (although of course, snakes don't have ears) as you curl your spine up and away from the ground. From an initial wide, far-forward position, your hands might creep closer as you gain strength and flexibility in the pose. A couple of folded blankets or yoga blocks under the front of the pelvis can work wonders, effectively 'making room' for your long arms and lessening any strain on the lower back. Rolling the heels away from each other such that the whole leg internally rotates from the hip socket will, for many bodies, create additional space and ease in the lower back.

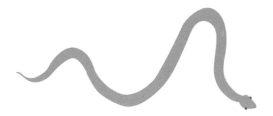

PIGEON POSE
Kapotasana/Eka Pada Rajakapotasana

....

THE PIGEON gives its name to two distinct poses (a forward and a backbend), each an elegant deconstruction of avian angles. In the forward-bending phase, the leading leg is deeply folded at the hip and bent at the knee, mimicking the elbow and wrist joints of a bird's wing, while the trailing leg stretches back like the long primary feathers, ending in the wing tip. The whole shape has a gorgeous resting lightness about it, albeit tempered by an often intense stretch across the back of the leading hip. When roused up out of its resting form into the backbend phase, the pose becomes a different bird altogether: a preening king pigeon with puffed-out chest and flirty tail feathers.

IN CONTEXT

The way you feel about pigeons is highly dependent on the place where you live. City-dwellers look at a pigeon and see a pest: a glassy-eyed rat with feathers. Out in the countryside, the same species of bird is fat and glossy with a comforting coo and a gift for slapstick. I often see one of them tumbling out of a tree in my garden after losing a squabble with its own legs. Their soft grey, blush pink and glossy green feathers would surely strike us as beautiful if they weren't so common in the UK.

In keeping with its rather ordinary namesake, the origins of *kapotasana* are not particularly ancient or religious. It isn't described in any of the older hatha yoga texts and it seems most likely that

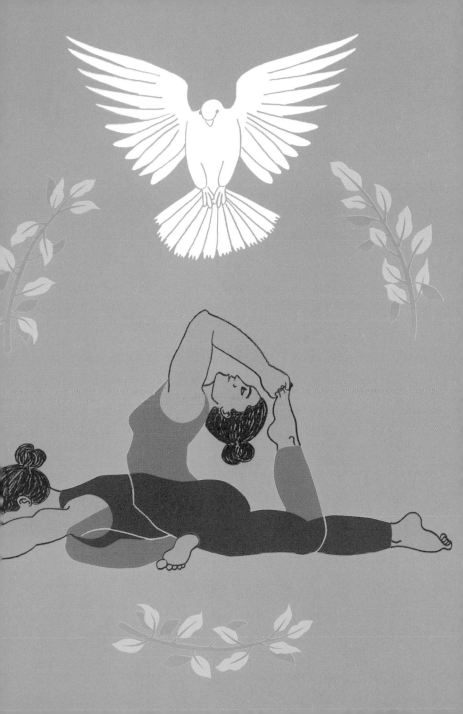

the pose entered the repertoire when hatha yoga began to evolve into its modern gymnastic phase, in the Mysore yoga schools of the 1930s–50s. As noted earlier, there's plenty of fascinating material to illustrate this period of intense cross-fertilisation between European gymnastics and Indian physical culture. In Mark Singleton's seminal 2010 work *Yoga Body*, he shares a photo of British gymnast Adonia Wallace from a 1935 issue of *Health and Strength* magazine. Billed as 'the Girl with the Perfect Figure', she demonstrates a stretching exercise identical to the one that B.K.S. Iyengar would later catalogue as *eka pada rajakapotasana* (literally, 'one-legged king pigeon pose').

Thus liberated from any particular religious or philosophical entanglements, perhaps we're freer than usual to bring our own interpretations and symbolism to the Pigeon pose. Here's one suggestion: bird bones are famously hollow, but you might be surprised to learn that it doesn't make them significantly lighter than mammal bones. However, they are denser, stiffer and stronger – all qualities that optimise them for flight. What's really extraordinary about the hollow spaces in a bird's bones is that some of them contain air sacs that help with oxygen intake and circulation during flight. In effect, these air sacs are an extension of the bird's lungs. That means its breathing system reaches all the way into its skeleton and takes up about a fifth of a bird's body, compared to only about one-twentieth of the average mammal's.

IN PRACTICE

This pose is unusual in that it combines forward and back bending under the same heading. Spinal flexion (forward bending) opens the back surface of the body by folding the head towards the feet or pelvis, usually with the aid of gravity. Spinal extension (back bending) opens the front surface of the body, usually by the combined effort of the muscles of the back and limbs. The mood of a forward bend tends to be more passive, calming, introverted, while backbends are energetically more active, stimulating and extroverted.

For the sake of argument, I'm going to call the two phases of pigeon pose 'Sleepy Pigeon' and 'Sexy Pigeon'. The forward-folded phase of Pigeon pose – Sleepy Pigeon – tends to lower your levels of reactivity and arousal. From a physiological point of view, Sleepy Pigeon expands the back surface of the ribcage and allows the heart to rest forwards away from the lungs, literally giving you more breathing space. Because putting your torso into a prone (face down) position allows you to access more of your available lung tissue and increases oxygenation of the blood, it's widely used in hospital care to help patients in respiratory distress – but all of us can benefit from it. To intensify your experience of this subtle change, imagine you have bird bones and each in-breath is perfusing your whole skeleton with energising oxygen. No need to make any extra effort to breathe, just let your inner bird enjoy the moment.

From this light, bird-boned headspace, moving into the active, back-bending phase of the pose may feel a little less effortful than usual. Along with its impressive lungs, a bird's heart is also relatively larger and more powerful than a mammal's. For a running animal like a human, physical strength is concentrated in the hips and legs; for a bird, by far the largest muscles in its body are the ones in its chest responsible for moving the wings. Male pigeons exaggerate their strength as part of mating displays by arching their backs, fluffing up their chest feathers and strutting like crazy. In the second, Sexy Pigeon phase of the pose, there's a sense of letting your chest puff proudly up and out as you gently push your hands into the ground and come into a backbend, supported on the bent leading leg and the front of the pelvis. The final refinement, if you're feeling both jaunty and well-balanced, is to raise the back foot like a tail feather and (carefully) reach around, or up and over, to take hold of your toes with one or both hands.

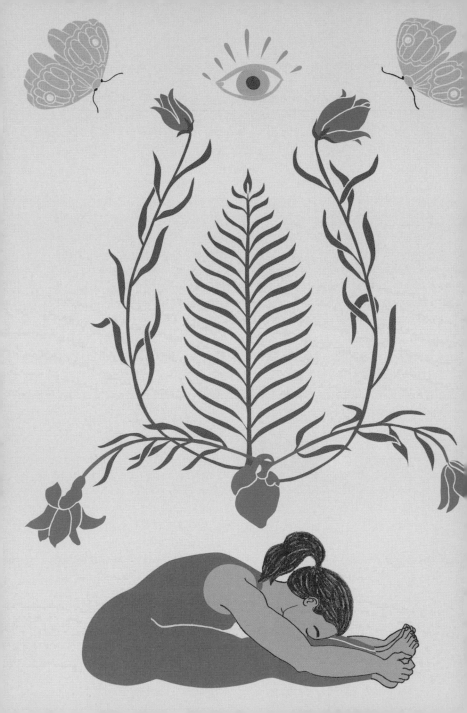

FORWARD FOLD
Paschimottanasana

....

ALL OF THE FORWARD-BENDING postures in yoga are variations on a simple theme: a hairpin bend at the hips that brings your forehead towards your knees. The oldest-known description of this pose, in the medieval *Hathayogapradipika*, calls it *paschimottanasana* – literally, 'west-side-extended pose', the west side of the body meaning the back. This version is performed seated, fingertips reaching to toes, but turned through 90 degrees to vertical, it's a standing forward bend (*uttanasana*); flipped through 180, it's the Plough pose (*halasana*). You start to see how those ancient scribes who boasted of 8.4 million yoga poses (or even just 84) might have been using some creative accounting: there are, after all, only so many ways to bend a human body.

IN CONTEXT

According to the *Hathayogapradipika*, this pose causes your *prana* or subtle energy to rise through the central channel, stokes your digestive fires, and flattens the belly. From an anatomical point of view, although we think of it as a back stretch, it actually tests the hip flexibility rather more than that of the spine. In order to execute a full 180-degree hairpin and lay your chest along your thighs, you'll need roughly 120 degrees of hip flexion, with the remaining 60-ish degrees of forward bend coming from the lumbar spine. That means lots of length is demanded of the hamstrings and hip flexor muscles in order to allow the pelvis to swivel forwards.

In the English-speaking West, we're obsessed with being able to touch our toes. From 1956–2012 (in other words, from Eisenhower to Obama), all public-school children in the US were supposed to benchmark themselves against a set of physical challenges known as the Presidential Fitness Test. Among the shuttle-runs and sit-ups was a flexibility test called the 'V-Seat Reach': the posture formerly known as *paschimottanasana*. Students were graded on how far they could reach towards or past their toes, from a straight-legged seated position.

So, is flexibility really a good test of fitness? Well, sometimes. In a study of 526 healthy adults, researchers from the University of North Texas found that among the over-40s in the group, prowess in the V-Seat Reach was strongly correlated with the flexibility of their cardiac arteries – one of the key elements of heart health. Stiffer arteries make the heart work much harder and may contribute to an increased risk of heart attack and stroke over time. There's also some accidental evidence to show that the relationship between hamstring and heart flexibility can be a positive one: another Texan study, this time at the University of Texas at Austin, was designed to explore whether weightlifting increased arterial stiffening. Although there was no change in the study group, the control group was assigned stretching exercises instead of weightlifting and their arterial pliability increased by more than 20 per cent in 13 weeks.

Regardless of their heart health, a lot of men cry foul at toe-touching as a measure of fitness: male bodies tend to struggle more with it than female ones, most likely because their hamstrings and hip flexors are shorter, bulkier and less flexible. There are, after all, important biological reasons why the female pelvis should be equipped with more flexible tendons and capable of a larger range of motion, built as it is to permit an actual baby to wriggle through. The toe-touch test also discriminates against people with comparatively shorter arms and longer legs, since you can't stretch your way past that particular genetic trait, whatever your sex. But the test persists, from P.E. class to military fitness drills. If you can't touch your damn toes, what are you even doing in gym shorts?

When you tell a stranger you teach yoga, there are really only two responses. If they are already a yoga student, they say, 'Oh really? What kind?' and the game of pigeonholing begins. If they aren't, they say, 'Gosh I could never do yoga, I can't even touch my toes!' with a self-deprecating laugh. I always explain that while prowess at the V-Seat Reach is not a prerequisite for yoga, it might be a side benefit of taking up the practice – but it generally doesn't convince. It makes me sad that yoga classes are still very much the province of self-selected bendy folks, while those whose shorter hamstrings could benefit so much from some west-side stretches are left on the sidelines.

IN PRACTICE

Those stats about hip versus lumbar flexibility might be helpful to remember. Lots of limbering and stretching work for the hips and hamstrings will set you up nicely for forward bending. It's no coincidence that teachers usually schedule seated forward bends towards the end of an *asana* class, when your body is nice and warm; don't expect this pose to come easy first thing on a winter's morning.

In the first stage of transition from upright seated to forward folding, it can help to envisage yourself lifting your abdominal organs up and out of the pelvis, then sending the tailbone and the pubic bone underneath right out behind you as you rotate the whole pelvis forwards. Once you've activated the maximum hip rotation available to you, it's time to recruit gravity to your aid. The weight of your head and shoulders moves forwards and down, arcing towards the shins. Don't recruit your arms to reach for the toes too soon: if you treat them as props not winches, you'll be able to ease forwards rather than drag yourself into the pose.

SQUAT
Utkatasana

....

THIS POSE IS SO SIMPLE that it hardly needs description, but here goes. From a standing position, fold your knees and hips to their fullest extent to bring the buttocks towards your heels.

Across most of the world, this is the default position for many sorts of work and all sorts of waiting. Whether you're running a market stall in Vietnam, hanging out at a bus stop in Kenya or milking a cow in India, chances are you'll be spending at least part of your time on your haunches.

IN CONTEXT

Squatting is a basic human movement that has become critically endangered by our chair-centric existence. At least, that's the contention of a vocal new movement of anti-chair activists who like to proclaim that 'sitting is the new smoking'. While I don't think that particular comparison holds water, they're definitely on to something. In societies where squatting is still widespread, people have been found to suffer much less from low back pain, constipation and haemorrhoids. In more industrialised parts of the world, we've reinvented squats as a butt-sculpting exercise and built multi-million-dollar industries around not just selling chairs but also treatments and remedies for – oh look, it's our old friends low back pain, constipation and haemorrhoids. Don't be fooled by the sinister machinations of Big Chair! All those comfy seating options are wrecking our nether regions, and it's time to stage a squat-in.

Sitting upright in a chair, with your legs at a roughly 90-degree angle to your spine, has become our paradigm for good posture. Yet

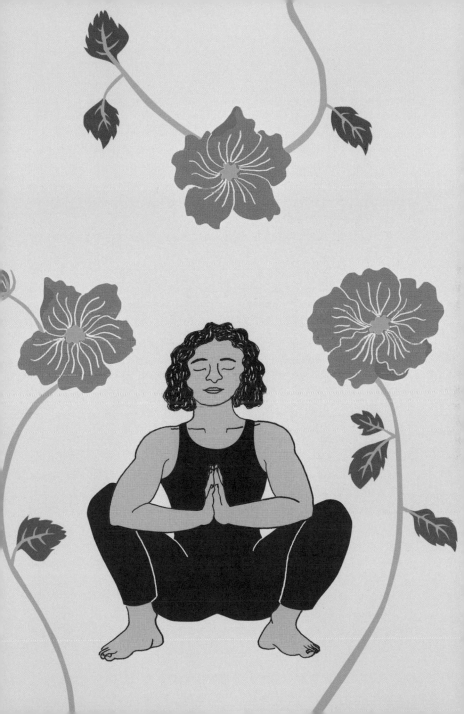

it's far from beneficial in the long term, especially given that many of us spend the lion's share of our waking hours in this shape. The musculature of your lower back is designed to support a lumbar curve; chair sitting flattens this curve, which means the low back muscles tend to get tight and strained over long periods. Standing desks help a lot, allowing the hips to move between the 90-degree angle and a 180-degree, straight-up-and-down position. But most of us rarely go much lower than 90 degrees, even though our hip joints are obviously adapted to allow us to fold our thighs right in towards the belly and rest there.

You might suppose that in a less chair-obsessed environment like, say, medieval India, squatting would be too ordinary an event to qualify as a yoga pose. Yet squatting *asana* appear in the *Yogashastra* of Hemachandra, tentatively dated to the eleventh century. *Utkatasana* is listed as a simple squatting pose with the buttocks touching the heels, while *godohikasana* – 'milking pose' – is the same posture with the heels off the ground (incidentally, you can still see Indian farmers squatting to milk their cows today). It's safe to assume that the practice described here was long-duration, endurance squatting, rather than the odd 30 seconds here and there: the commentary goes on to say that the squatting pose is taught because it's practised by certain Jain monks as part of an intensive course of austerity. At any rate, I'd say it's a mistake to think that everyone in pre-modern India was totally comfortable hanging out in a squat all day; you can therefore feel much better about finding it torturous too.

So, why squat? For one, your rectum will thank you. Chair sitting – or indeed toilet sitting – puts an unhelpful kink in the pipes and stagnant bowels are bad news. Some unlucky researchers X-rayed people using sitting versus squatting toilets, and concluded the latter is a much more ergonomic solution for throughput. Outside of the bathroom, the reduced hip and back mobility that results from a sedentary lifestyle affects all aspects of movement as you get older. Joint range of motion works on a fairly unforgiving 'use it or lose it' model: the sooner we start reactivating the full spectrum of natural movement available to us, the better.

IN PRACTICE

Toddlers squat with complete ease. It's one of those natural abilities that we grow out of, thanks to the ubiquity of chairs – but most of us can get back at least some facility once we rehabilitate our squatting muscles. It's common to experience discomfort at first, particularly if you try to stay still – remember the Jain monks, squatting to prove their indifference to the illusion of physical reality? Eleventh-century yogins were very much concerned with discipline, but if your primary goal is range of motion, then it makes sense to move within the squat shape. Feet together, feet apart. Toes parallel, or turned out. Heels high, low, or resting on a rolled mat. Spine in deep flexion, like a tortoise shell, or more extended. Try keeping your balance while you lower one knee, then the other. Move back and forth between a squat and a standing forward bend, or between a squat and a high kneeling position with toes tucked under. These are creepy-crawly, monkey sort of movements, keeping your centre of gravity low to the ground. As you explore and begin to internalise these unfamiliar patterns, keep in mind that you're reclaiming movements that are your mammalian birthright.

The squat is a great example of a pose that should – and easily can – wriggle its way off the yoga mat and into your everyday life. A little creative rearranging of the furniture will help: for example, you could try floor cushions in front of the TV or an office chair with a wide enough seat that you can squat on top of it. If they're not already common in your area, installing a squatting toilet might feel like a step too far; luckily, a simple foot-rest in front of the throne can work minor miracles.

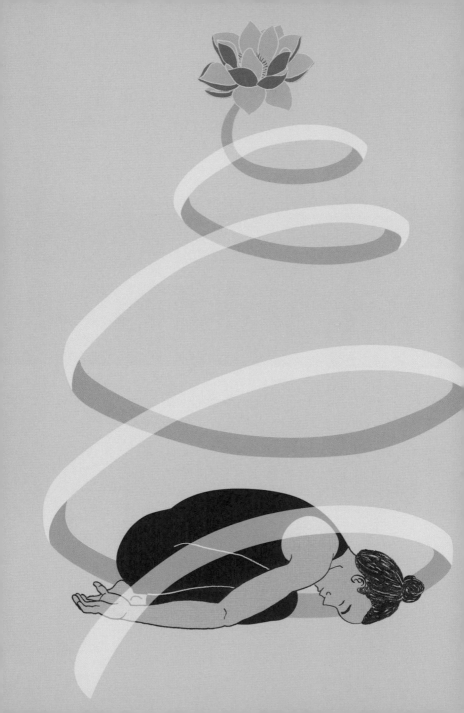

CHILD'S POSE
Balasana

....

From a kneeling position, keeping the hips settled on the heels, fold forwards from the hips and rest your forehead on the ground (if it reaches) or on a suitable prop or cushion. This is *balasana*, the pose of the child.

IN CONTEXT

Yoga *asana* (the 'curious poses' for which this book is named) are just one of eight different practices deemed essential to the goal of yoga. Often called the 'eight limbs', which sounds a little spidery, they are more precisely defined as 'adjuncts' or 'auxiliaries': all eight must be put to work in cooperation in order to achieve the ultimate goal of yoga. The first two 'limbs' make up the moral code of yoga: five *yamas* or moral duties (non-violence, truthfulness, not stealing, chastity and not being acquisitive) and five *niyamas*: restraints or observances (cleanliness, contentment, self-discipline, study and devotion to a higher power). Put together, these rules of conduct should ensure that students of yoga don't behave like assholes. With that locked down, we can proceed to *asana*, then *pranayama* – breath control exercises.

The next of the eight prerequisites for yoga is *pratyahara*: the withdrawal of the senses from their external objects. This drawing inwards of the mind, away from the outside world and towards itself, is the turning point between the first four practices (which interact with outward, physical reality), and the last three, introspective ones (*dharana*, *dhyana* and *samadhi* – progressive states of meditative absorption that take place in the realm of consciousness alone). Sense withdrawal is a key skill for the would-be yogi to develop because the yoga system posits that to master the mind, we must first restrain the senses that feed us such distractingly vivid impressions of the world around us. While the mind is busy interpreting all the things we can see, feel, hear, taste and smell, it will always be subject to fluctuations and deluded as to its true nature.

Child's pose is a great way to get a taste for this inward turn. If you tuck your face in towards your knees and close your eyes, it's easy to pull your attention inside, too. Like a tortoise retreating into its shell, the rigid structure of the back ribs provides shelter for all your squishy, vulnerable bits.

When my son was very young, he would sometimes adopt this position during a game of hide and seek, pulling his clothes up over his head to make it dark. On the basis that 'if I can't see you, you can't see me', this is a totally legitimate hiding place for a two-year-old, even if to an untrained eye he's hard to miss, on full display in the middle of the living room carpet in *Spider-Man* pyjamas. And it's really difficult not to play along: I never did 'find' him when he did this, so the ploy worked.

There is something slightly magical about disappearing into Child's pose. It sends a very clear 'do not disturb' signal to the world at large. For most of us, although by no means for all, it feels safe to rest here: withdrawn, a little regressed, in your tortoise shell.

An image that helps me even more than the tortoise is that of a sea anemone. I like to visualise my senses as thousands of delicate, hypersensitive tendrils, wafting gently as they detect microscopic food particles in the ocean currents. When it's time to withdraw, my mind-urchin can fold each tendril back in on itself in an instant, pulling all that squirming curiosity out of the ocean and into the black-velvet silence of its rigid exoskeleton. It's simultaneously a contraction and a relaxation. Everything that was attuned to the vast space around me fits neatly into the bounded space within me and becomes still.

IN PRACTICE

In Child's pose, there's a sense of wrapping the body protectively around its soft centre. You'll recall the image of the lotus room inside the heart that I touched on in the section about Hero pose (*see also* p. 17). Here, the heart lotus is hidden in the centre of the pose, like a dazzling jewel inside a Fabergé egg. Hugging the heart close in this way can be a lovely, self-soothing gesture. To this act of metaphorical self-care we could add the benefits of a humble ego: this forward bend is culturally encoded as a gesture of submission and devotion, as in *I bow at your feet*.

What emotions does that idea arouse in you? If your reaction is that you don't want that attitude in your emotional vocabulary, then I sympathise: I was not raised by my feminist mentors to see submission as a virtue. I'm particularly allergic to the idea of submitting to individual human authority, whether it's exerted by a charismatic yoga teacher or a strict parent. But how exhausting, never to surrender! And how hard to grow old without ever having exercised that emotional muscle. Because surrender overcomes all of us, in the end: in the face of grief and loss, or physical infirmity, or the vagaries of circumstance. Life is constantly reminding us we're not really in charge. In the words of Grateful Dead roadie Big Steve Parish (no stranger to entropy and chaos), 'The situation is the boss'. By practising surrender, we learn the art of yielding when we have no option – like a sapling that bends in the face of a storm, rather than breaking.

The discipline of *pratyahara*, withdrawal of the senses from their objects, is itself a form of surrender. It's a letting down of your guard as you consciously notice each of your senses and turn them inwards, away from their usual roles as the highly reactive gatekeepers to your nervous system. But relinquishing the attempt to predict or control the external environment opens up new possibilities for sensing your internal one.

As you rest in Child's pose, if it feels safe and comfortable for you, you might like to try sensing each layer of your body from the outside in. First, become aware of the whole outline of your shape, the amount of space you take up in the surrounding air. Next, slowly move inwards, through a complex folded puzzle of bones and muscles, then on into the softness of your internal organs, coming to rest inside the heart. When you're ready, move your attention out through the layers again and maybe even beyond your physical outline to see if you can extend those invisible sea urchin sense tentacles into the space around you, before uncurling your physical body and bringing your face back to the world.

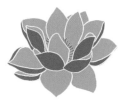

HAPPY BABY POSE
Ananda Balasana

....

SOME YOGA POSES are fierce and powerful; others are graceful and elegant. Some have a profound stillness and calm about them – and then there's the Happy Baby.

To get into the baby groove, lie down on your back and bend your knees in towards your chest. Reach both arms in between your legs and grasp the outsides of each foot with the same-side hand. Orient the soles of your feet towards the ceiling, and, well, roll around a bit. It's the flip side of Child's pose (p. 141), with the attitude to match: exploratory and playful, rather than introspective and still.

IN CONTEXT

Ananda balasana – 'blissful baby' – is not a traditional yoga *asana*. It's a modern name for an effective, if not particularly elegant, warm-up/cool-down exercise that can provide a lovely stretch for all sorts of muscles around the hips, pelvis and hamstrings. This pose is well named, not just because lots of babies really do love doing this, but because it tends to tip you into a sort of giggly, zoned-out baby state almost immediately. It's just not possible to maintain whatever adult masks you usually wear – dynamic professional, respected member of the community, wise parent – while holding your toes and rocking on your back like a drunken beetle.

Human babies are rather underdeveloped compared to most of our mammalian cousins. If you've ever seen a lamb or foal being born, you'll know that healthy newborn quadrupeds are generally able to stand up within the first half hour. It takes most humans about a year to get to that stage. We arrive in the world as helpless, wriggling grubs, equipped with a few unconscious reflexes to help us feed and attract attention. An extended period of intense physical and mental development ensues: we must first gain control of our muscles and coordinate the movement of our limbs, and then figure out how to negotiate with gravity as we make the transition from four- to two-limbed perambulation. We achieve this not through study or structured training, but through play – the first and purest form of empirical science.

Experimenting with our bodily movements, with gravity, with the world around us and its sensory inputs: in our early years, learning is play and vice versa. The only way for a baby to become more effective in the world is to try stuff out and see what happens. We kick and flex, arch our spines, grasp with our hands, taste everything we can reach. Little by little, the involuntary movements come under our conscious control.

As it happens, the concept of play is central to Indian philosophy. The Sanskrit word *lila* can mean play, sport, drama or spontaneity: something joyous and creative, free from purpose or consequences. It's a divine quality, because of that very freedom. Of all the gods, Krishna is perhaps the most devoted to such games. Even as a baby, his divine nature reveals itself through a series of mischievous escapades. One earns him the nickname 'Butter Thief' after he steals a whole pat of freshly churned butter and shares it with the monkeys. In another episode, he is out in the fields playing with the cowherds' children when he decides to taste some mud (we've all met that kid). One of his friends runs off to tell Krishna's foster-mother Yashoda, who has not yet recognised that there's something atypical about the blue-skinned, freakishly strong toddler. Of course, Krishna shakes his head vigorously in denial, but she insists that he should open his mouth to prove there is no mud inside. The little god eventually capitulates. To Yashoda's horror, she looks inside his mouth to see not baby teeth, tonsils and dirt, but the whole of the universe: orbiting planets, the

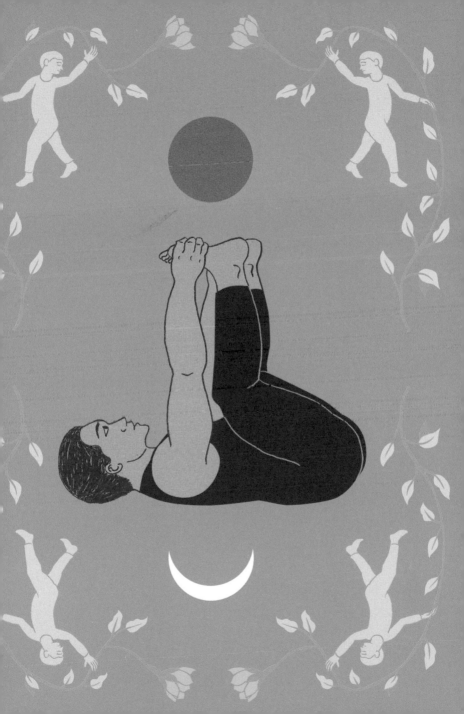

Earth with its vast oceans and towering mountains, velvet-black heavens studded with stars, the wind and the lightning, and the very elements themselves. In that moment, she finally realises that Krishna is a god.

For some schools of Indian thought, the whole material universe is the product of divine play: it is *maya lila*, an illusion created by the playful expansion of pure consciousness. Although largely indifferent to the fates of the mortals caught up in its fictions, this game is not exactly irresponsible in the normal sense. It's just that it takes place on a plane where responsibility is a meaningless concept. The rules of cause and effect are for mere mortals to grapple with. From this viewpoint, being a god is a lot like being a baby: you're free to give full rein to your curiosity and innocent of any reasons to hold back.

But human babies have to grow up. As you mature, each tiny encounter with the big world adds to your body's growing library of notes, limitations and risk assessments, making your physical interactions with the world ever so slightly more complex and fraught, day by day. In yogic terms, you become more weighed down by the build-up of *karma* and further removed from pure bliss, pure play. So what would it feel like to re-engage with your physical experience from this place of 'blissful baby'? A bit like a stage actor, thoroughly invested in your role in the drama but free from any real-world outcomes.

IN PRACTICE

I think the yoga mat is a fantastic place to experiment with being a baby-god for a while (the office, not so much). Happy Baby pose reminds me to keep an element of playful curiosity in my yoga practice. It's easy to take yoga too seriously. Amid the systematic training and 'this pose is for this purpose' and endless alignment cues and prohibitions, I want to remember to make room for 'let's try it out and see what happens'.

7
LYING DOWN

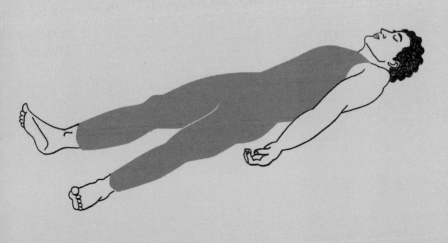

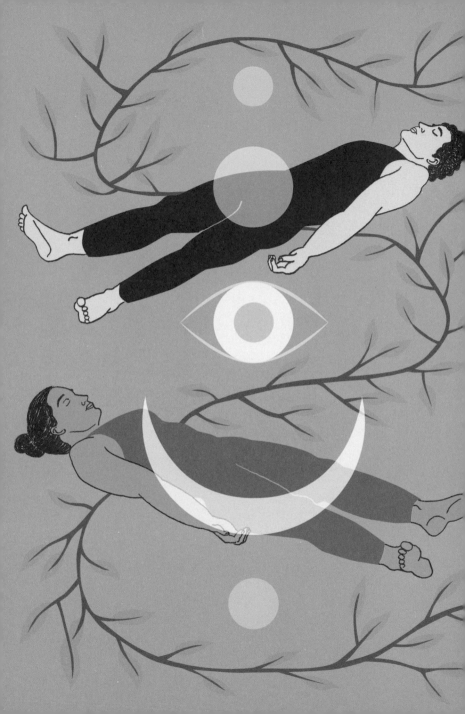

CORPSE POSE
Shavasana

....

BACK WHEN I WAS STUDYING to become a yoga teacher, I taught my first ever class with an assessor looking on. I got all the way through to the final five minutes and was starting to congratulate myself on a hurdle successfully cleared. Beginner yoga teachers will relate to that moment of intense relief when all the students are finally lying down, flat on their backs, eyes closed. But my reprieve was short-lived: a schoolboy passing by the ground-floor studio windows peered in and shouted, loudly for comic effect, 'Oh my GOD, they're all DEAD!'

There are basically two options for yoga teachers when the outside world rudely intervenes during a quiet bit of class: acknowledge and make light of it, or flat-out ignore it. Inexperienced teachers tend to take the latter course, so I simply pretended it hadn't happened. With hindsight, I should have congratulated the students afterwards on the authenticity of their *shavasana*: Corpse pose.

IN CONTEXT

Among the disparate and often conflicting ambitions of hatha yoga devotees down the centuries, one has remained constant: the secret hope that this might be a technology for cheating death. In the foundational texts of pre-modern yoga, the advertised benefits seem clear. For example, the *Hathayogapradipika* tells us that when *kundalini* is awakened and all the chakras are opened, 'then indeed *sushumna* becomes the pathway of prana, mind is free of all connections and death is averted'. *HYP 3:3*

The fantasy of immortality is echoed in the seductive promises of modern wellness yoga, where denial of ageing, sickness and death hangs as thick in the air as the vaporised essential oil blends. In this fragrant world, the ideal yoga body never ages: it is as lithe as a teenager's and as flexible as a toddler's. It can be rejuvenated by chakra meditations and purified by inversions, and if it breaks or fails then it's on you for letting the bad vibes in. Those of us who grew up in the twentieth and twenty-first centuries have all internalised these messages to some extent because they're key verses in the gospel of late capitalism. If I can just work hard enough, eat the right 'clean' foods, make my body hard and beautiful enough, amass enough followers, maybe nothing bad will happen to me. Maybe I won't have to get old, get sick, or die.

But when the yogic texts talk of 'conquering death', is this actually what they mean?

There are two vital pieces of background to bring into the frame here. First, consider hatha yoga's roots in tantra, a set of ritual practices that proliferated in India and beyond between 500 and 1200 CE. Tantric techniques are much concerned with cultivating an intimacy with death in order to prepare for the death of the individual consciousness and rebirth as a *jivan-mukta*: a person 'liberated in this life'. Some Indian ascetic sects believed (and still believe) in the special symbolic power of meditating in cemeteries. Seated on or near a corpse, confronted with the physical reality of his existence, the yogin can burn away the ego-consciousness that holds him back from liberation, along with his fear of death. It's one among many tantric exercises in working with opposites, cultivating equanimity, and rising above the petty preoccupations of conventional morality.

A second important piece of context here is the doctrine of reincarnation. Indian spirituality takes as one of its foundational principles the concept of *maya*, cosmic illusion. This mysterious process creates and destroys the universe endlessly, necessitating the cyclical return of mortal existences and the accrual of *karma* –

until such time as our souls are enlightened and step beyond the illusion of human experience and into the reality of the absolute. Life (and death) on Earth is a suffering to be endured, over and over, unless you can attain liberation through spiritual practice – through yoga. A yogin conquers death by dissolving into pure consciousness and stepping off the hamster wheel of *karma*, not by prolonging his earthly days.

So, a corpse in the context of yoga is not something to be avoided. Immortality is achieved not by avoiding death, but by going *through* it: by the death of the personality, via the ritual initiations of yoga. It's not about maintaining your teenage figure, but rather gaining such radical acceptance of the impermanence of your ageing body that you can look death square in the face and smile. This is not to say that yoga makes it easy. Death doesn't suddenly stop being sad or scary, even when you convince yourself it's just a doorway to something better. For me, the message of Corpse pose is that some day, I'm going to have to stop running away from it – so I might as well get in some practice.

IN PRACTICE

Whatever your culture of origin, death is a heavy topic. If you go into the final relaxation stage of your yoga practice with a headful of existential questions, you're definitely going to overthink it. I may be a staunch defender of intellectual curiosity when it comes to yoga, but I'm also very clear that there's a certain point of yoga practice beyond which intellect tends to get in the way.

The ways of knowing that yoga philosophy offers are subtle and complex, and can't be reached through reason or enquiry alone. The final three 'limbs' of classical yoga are collectively known as *samyama*. This three-stage process starts with *dharana*, concentration: the holding of an idea or object of enquiry in mind until the white noise of the subconscious falls away and the object is completely understood in a way that transcends language or thought. Next comes *dhyana*, meditation: in this stage, the idea or object magically becomes part of the meditator. Finally, we reach *samadhi*, absorption: now the meditator and the object of meditation are not just in tune, but identical. Through these subtle stages of yoga, out beyond the intellectual realm, the practitioner has the experience of being at one with the idea.

Central to these kinds of knowing is a profound stillness: just as every action creates *karma*, so the cessation of activity clears away impediments to true understanding. If you can be still enough, there is no need to think: the truth will reveal itself in its own time.

Sometimes, teachers will tell you that the final resting pose is an opportunity to absorb the effects of the class. This is true: the feeling of having worked hard at yoga is distinctive, and wonderful, and worth wallowing in. Having spent some time in careful, deliberate movement and stillness, having stretched and balanced and strengthened and twisted, this is a moment to simply be, in a state of attention. There's a sense that all the poses that went before were just leading up to this moment: to the fleeting experience of not running away from what is.

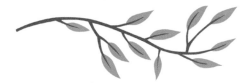

AFTERWORD

....

ALL THESE TANGLED THREADS of yoga, all this beautiful, infuriating complexity: it's a lot to take in. It's certainly a lot more than I was expecting when I looked at the tiny spider spinning its web on my yoga pose and idly wondered what on earth I was doing in that forward bend. I think I was hoping that at the end of yoga lay 'The Answer', and that with my machete of dogged enquiry I could hack away at the undergrowth and find the one path that would lead me straight there. But with a system – or an array of related systems – as ancient and complex as yoga, there's never a single, simple answer.

If, like me, you're a cultural and intellectual descendent of Plato and Saint Augustine (rather than, say, Lao Tse or the authors of the Upanishads), your basic thinking apparatus is trained around a dialectical model. In our system of thought, understanding is more or less the same thing as certainty: it comes only after you have tested and eliminated all the wrong answers, thereby logically proving the right one. Although it's a highly effective set of tools for enquiry, providing the basis for both the scientific method and the adventures of Sherlock Holmes, it turns out that other toolsets are available. But because this particular either/or way of sorting out the truth feels so natural to me, it can be deeply discombobulating to abandon it in favour of both/and.

That's what yoga asks of us, again and again: to hold several conflicting truths in mind. It insists that we recognise the kinship of opposites, seeing 'soft' and 'strong', 'minutely small' and 'infinitely large', not as opposite ends of a spectrum, but conjoined faces of the same coin. And it insists that we enter into this both/and experience, not just in the intellectual realm but with our whole bodies. In a culture that prizes certainty, ambiguity can be a deeply uncomfortable space to occupy, but the rewards for learning to tolerate or even thrive in it are profound.

Modern yoga practitioners must learn to juggle these two truths, for starters: that although each of us has a singular experience of yoga, yoga itself is plural. It's baked into Indian philosophy that *all* perception is a form of illusion; once you allow that concept to really land, then the existence of multiple answers to every yoga question may be a little easier to handle. You can go ahead and give up on the goal of nailing down the one true story, or the real authentic yoga.

Mind you, that doesn't mean that everyone's interpretation of yoga is equally valid: on the contrary, I believe we have a moral duty to apply discerning judgement to the stories we hear; to recognise the motivation behind each storyteller's account, tease out historical fact from fiction and bring as much clarity to the party as we are able. Because while it's right to recognise that yoga means many different things to different people, it's also right to have a well-founded sense of what it means to *you*.

One thing I am sure of is that the stories will continue to proliferate. The harder I strive to pursue my quest for The Answer, the denser the tangle seems to grow; the glow of enlightenment is always receding, just beyond reach. That's all part of the game, the *lila* that pulls us into the spinning dance of being human. Yet through the weeds, from time to time I catch a glancing view of something profoundly simple, as clear and irresistible as water. Something that might slake my intrinsic thirst for clarity and truth: that insatiable drive identified in the *Upanishads* as the soul's longing for itself.

In the thirteenth-century *Dattatreyayogashastra*, the earliest text to describe a system of yoga called *hatha*, the prescription is already clear: 'If diligent, through practice everyone, even the young or the old or the diseased, gradually obtains success in yoga. [...] Success happens for he who performs the practices – how could it happen for one who does not? [...] The wearing of religious garb does not bring success, nor does talking about it. Practice alone is the cause of success.'

Yoga at the individual level is a deeply introverted practice: a journey into the interior. Once you take that inward turn, you are on your own, with all the comforts and all the terrors that solitude brings. It's a great adventure, which holds out the promise of a great reward. We adopt these curious poses, learn some of the breath work, maybe the concentration and meditation practices too – and with patience, each of us finds the way to some inner spring, some sloping bank where we can slip silently into the water and become transparent, fluid, fundamental, even just for a moment. Maybe it's the one story we can never explain or articulate, and maybe that's all right.

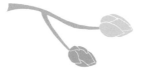

REFERENCES

MIGHTY POSE (p. 51)

NAIR, M. (2014) 'The Guru with a Stick', *Times of India*, https://bit.ly/tgwastoi

HEADSTAND (p. 91)

BROAD, WILLIAM J. (2012), *The Science of Yoga*, (New York: Simon & Schuster)

PEACOCK POSE (p. 95)

MALLINSON, J. and SINGLETON M. (trans.) (2017), *Roots of Yoga* (London: Penguin)

UPWARD-FACING BOW POSE (p. 115)

NAIR, S., SAGAR, M., et al. (2015), 'Do slumped and upright postures affect stress responses? A randomized trial', *Health Psychol.*, 34(6):632–41. DOI: 10.1037/hea0000146

STREETER, C. C., GERBARG, P. L., et al. (2020), *The Journal of Alternative and Complementary Medicine*, 190–197. DOI: 10.1089/acm.2019.0234

COBRA POSE (p. 123)

University of Melbourne, 'Snakebite in India', https://bit.ly/UoMISP

SURAWEERA, W., WARRELL, D. et al. (2020), 'Trends in snakebite deaths in India from 2000 to 2019 in a nationally representative mortality study', *eLife* https://elifesciences.org/articles/54076

BERTELS, J., BOURGUIGNON, M. et al. (2020), 'Snakes elicit specific neural responses in the human infant brain', *Nature* https://www.nature.com/articles/s41598-020-63619-y

PIGEON POSE (p. 128)

EHRLICH, P., DOBKIN, D. S., and WHEYE, D. (1988), 'Adaptations for Flight' https://stanford.io/3vbRpjH

ALBERT R.K., HUBMAYR R.D. (2000), 'The prone position eliminates compression of the lungs by the heart', *Am J Respir Crit Care Med*, 161(5):1660-5. DOI: 10.1164/ajrccm. 161.5.9901037

HENDERSON, W. R., GRIESDALE, D. E. G. et al., (2014),

'Does prone positioning improve oxygenation and reduce mortality in patients with acute respiratory distress syndrome?', *Can Respir J.*, 2014 21(4): 213–215. DOI: 10.1155/2014/472136

LANSFORD, R. and RUGONYI, S. (2020), 'Follow Me! A Tale of Avian Heart Development with Comparisons to Mammal Heart Development', *J Cardiovasc Dev Dis.*, 7(1): 8. DOI: 10.3390/jcdd7010008

FORWARD FOLD (*p. 133*)

YAMAMOTO, K., KAWANO, H. et al. (2009), 'Poor trunk flexibility is associated with arterial stiffening', *Am J Physiol Heart Circ Physiol*, 297(4):H1314-8. DOI: 10.1152/ajpheart.00061.2009

CORTEZ-COOPER, M. Y., ANTON, M. M. (2007), 'The effects of strength training on central arterial compliance in middle-aged and older adults', Department of Kinesiology and Health Education, The University of Texas at Austin, Texas, USA. DOI: 10.1.1.495.5470

SQUAT (*p. 136*)

SAKAKIBARA R., TSUNOYAMA K. et al. (2010), 'Influence of Body Position on Defecation in Humans' *Low Urin Tract Symptoms,* 2(1):16-21.. DOI: 10.1111/j.1757-5672.2009.00057.x

AFTERWORD (*p. 155*)

MALLINSON, J. and SINGLETON M. (trans.) (2017), *Roots of Yoga* (London: Penguin)

FURTHER READING

BLACKABY, P. (2020), *Intelligent Yoga* (Leicester: Matador)

COULTER, H. DAVID (2010), *Anatomy of Hatha Yoga,* (Honesdale, PA: Body & Breath)

DESIKACHAR, T.K.V. (1999), *The Heart of Yoga* (Rochester, VT: Inner Traditions)

IYENGAR, B.K.S. (2015), *Light on Yoga* (New York: Thorsons)

NAGEL, THOMAS (1974), 'What is it like to be a bat?', *The Philosophical Review*, 83(4): 43--450. www.jstor.org/stable/2183914

SWAMI PUROHIT and YEATS, W. B. (1975), *The Ten Principal Upanishads* (London: Faber)

SRI SWAMI SATCHIDANANDA (trans.) (2012), *The Yoga Sutras of Patanjali* (Buckingham, VT: Integral Yoga Publications)

SINGLETON, MARK (2010), *Yoga Body,* (Oxford: OUP)

SWAMI MUKTIBODHANANDA (2000), *Hathayogapradipika* (Bihar: Yoga Publications Trust)

ACKNOWLEDGEMENTS

....

LET ME START where every student of yoga must: with the deepest bow of thanks to my teachers. Foremost among those is Tara Fraser, whose wisdom has illuminated my past 15 years of yoga studies. Also James Jewell (for outdoor yoga with the guru-spider, and so much more) and Kevin Walker (for the basement ashtanga that started it all). Behind these individuals stand all the generations before them: all the patient, generous sharers of yoga traditions and innovations. I owe them a great debt of gratitude; with this book, I hope I can begin to pay it forward.

The seed for Curious Poses was planted and nurtured by Zoë Blanc, my amazing editor. It was her initial suggestion for me to write a book about yoga postures, and our subsequent conversations were invaluable in giving shape and direction to my ideas. I'm grateful for both her impeccable taste and judgement, and her unwavering support. The whole team at Green Tree has been a joy to work with; from the outset, they completely 'got' the book and built it into something more than I could ever have hoped for.

Amanda León's lush, evocative illustrations brilliantly capture the intentions of the text and add richness and texture to the experience of reading it. I am very fortunate to have found an illustrator whose talent and sensibility fit the book so perfectly.

Finally, to my partner, Justin, and my son, Thomas, by turns cheerleaders, pit crew and joyful distraction through the long pandemic months of writing and editing: thank you. I love you immeasurably.